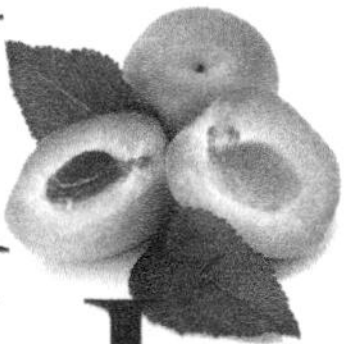

JOSEPH SMITH AND NATURAL FOODS

JOSEPH SMITH

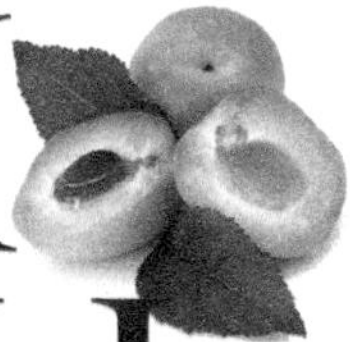

AND NATURAL FOODS

JOHN HEINERMAN

BONNEVILLE BOOKS

SPRINGVILLE, UTAH

ISBN 13: 978-1-55517-503-0
v.2

Published by Bonneville Books, an imprint of Cedar Fort, Inc., 2373 W. 700 S., Springville, UT 84663
Distributed by Cedar Fort, Inc., www.cedarfort.com

Cover design by Jen Boss
Cover design © 2009 by Lyle Mortimer
Typeset by Virginia Reeder

Printed in the United States of America

10 9 8 7 6 5 4 3 2 1

Printed on acid-free paper

To:

Jacob and Joseph Heinerman, who believe in the natural ways of living and eating right.

ACKNOWLEDGMENTS

The author is grateful for the help of his father and brother, Jacob and Joseph Heinerman, and the assistance they rendered in providing him with clues and suggestions. Also, to his good friend, Dee Mar Brower, for his unfailing support and constant encouragement in so detailed a work. Special consideration is likewise given the young lady of unnamed source at the University of Utah Western Americana section, who so thoughtfully referred the author to an account book located in their archives which was the source of much valuable information for certain sections of this book. Grateful mention also goes to Mr. and Mrs. Howard Stevens of Mapleton, Utah, for their kind loan of certain books, pamphlets, and magazine articles. And, finally, heartfelt appreciation is extended to Him who makes "the pen mightier than the sword."

Table of Contents

A thorough reformation is needed in regard to our eating and drinking.

—Brigham Young
(Journal of Discourses 12:192)

If we wish to raise a healthy, noble-looking, intellectual and perfect race of men and women, we must feed our children properly.

—George Q. Cannon
(Journal of Discourses 12:223)

INTRODUCTION

This study has been done more for human interest reasons than for scientific purposes. The author, however, is no layman in terms of the food business. He has worked in the restaurant trade for the approximate space of seven years or more, and is well acquainted with the subjects about which he is writing. But his treatment of them involves people more than facts, souls more than statistics. It would be closer to the truth to say that this is a history of the Mormon people and their food. Diet alone is not the subject in discussion. The mouths and faces behind what is being consumed or sold is likewise given an equal share of investigative interest.

This approach has been necessary because of the dearth of material which exists upon the subject of food among the Mormon pioneers. Not everyone, you know, kept an accurate record of what they ate and drank. That is one of the more insignificant things in one's life to be recorded, and, as such, held little regard for worthy entry into most diaries and journals of that time. However, with the sparse amount of information available and a little help from the right source, plus the human element involved, an intriguing and fascinating work has been put together, that will, in the end, serve the purpose for which it was written: to satisfy the spiritual and temporal appetites of the true history gourmet, and establish once and for all the definite fact, in an age of artificial nutrition, that Joseph Smith and his people believed in and ate NATURAL FOODS of the earth.

—The Author

February 15, 1976

Manti, Utah

CHAPTER ONE

SPOT OF TEA

(Joseph Smith and Herbal Drinks)

Whenever the British find themselves wanting for a break or temporary refreshment, they generally pause for what is termed in their peculiar venacular "a spot of tea." From such a moment of pleasant diversion, they obtain much-needed relief and relaxation from the pressing matters which they might, at that time, happen to be engaged in. Though basically psychological, it achieves for them the same results that the favorite American "coffee break" does for us over here.

At one time, in our nation's illustrious past, the tea business happened to be quite the thing, though. As early as the beginning of the 1800s, the traffic and trade in this certain commodity excelled even what the ordinary history buffs suppose it may have been. The plant was Ginseng, the product was tea, and the customer was faraway China.

> *History and science have their romances as vivid and as fascinating as any in the realms of fiction. No story ever told has surpassed in interest the history of this mysterious plant Ginseng, the root that for nearly 200 years has been an important article of export to China.*
>
> *Until a few years ago not one in a hundred intelligent Americans living in cities and towns ever heard of the plant, and those in the wilder parts of the country who dug and sold the roots could tell nothing of its history and use. Their fore-fathers had dug and sold Ginseng. They merely followed the old custom.*
>
> *The natural range of Ginseng growing wild in the United States is north to the Canadian line, embracing all the states of Maine, New Hampshire, Vermont, Massachusetts, Connecticut, Rhode Island, Delaware, New York, Pennsylvania, New Jersey, Maryland, Ohio, West Virginia, Indiana, Illinois, Michigan, Wisconsin, Kentucky and Tennessee. It is also found in a greater part of the following states: Minnesota, Iowa,*

Missouri, North and South Carolina, Georgia and Alabama. Until recently the plant was found growing wild in the above states in abundance, especially those states touched by the Allegheny Mountains. The plant is also found in Ontario and Quebec, Canada, but has become scarce there also, owing to persistent hunting. It also grows sparingly in the states west of and bordering on the Mississippi River.

Ginseng in the United States was not considered of any medicinal value until about 1905, but in China it is and has been highly prized for medicinal purposes and large quantities of the root are exported to that country. [1]

The story behind the development of this unusual commerce with China, is, in itself, a remarkable tale:

Our native ginseng first came to the attention of Europeans when Father Joseph Lafitau, who had been a missionary in China, recognized the similar American plant growing near a Mohawk village in Canada. He set up ovens and had the Mohawks gather and cure ginseng for the Chinese market. By 1717, it was being brought from as far away as Green Bay, Wisconsin, by the Fox Indians, and shipped to Hong Kong via France. In 1783, the Empress of China sailed for Macao with a load of ginseng to exchange for tea, ginger, silk and camphor. Also in 1784, George Washington wrote, "In passing through the mountains, I met a number of persons and pack horses going over the mountain with ginseng." In 1793, Andre' Michaux wrote that ginseng was the only product of Kentucky that could be transported overland to Philadelphia.

By 1798, John Drayton of South Carolina said, "It is so much sought after by the Cherokees for trade it is by no means as plentiful as it used to be in this state." Ginseng gathered had begun to be a way of life for many pioneers. A man could go "sang hunting" and return with a fortune; or in those perilous times, might never return at all.

The early colonists not only gathered ginseng for sale, but used it in tea to encourage the appetite or strengthen the digestion, especially of elderly persons or puny children. Ginseng plus black cherry and yellowroot made a potent tonic, especially with the addition of some homemade whiskey. An early herbal suggested gathering ginseng root and steeping it with chamomile flowers for fainting females.

Colonel Byrd, in his History of the Dividing Line, wrote, "To help cure fatigue, I used to chew a root of ginseng as I walked along. This kept up my spirits. It gives an uncommon warmth and vigor to the blood. It cheers the heart of a man that has a bad wife, and makes him look down with great composure upon the crosses of the world. It will make old age amiable by rendering it lively, cheerful and good-humored." Many early settlers dug ginseng roots for their own use and never thought of selling it. By 1800, several patent medicines on the market featured "seng" or "sangtone."

With some domestic sale, as well as a continuing foreign market, "sanging" became a business in the rick deciduous forests of the American heartland, and on the slopes of the Catskills, the Poconos, the Alleghenies, and the Appalachians.

It was inevitable that some would try to cash in on such a profitable and easy crop by cultivating it. Thus there was a craze for ginseng gardens from 1889 through 1905, with centers in Amberg, Wisconsin, and Chardon, Ohio. Later New York state and then Michigan became the centers of ginseng production. Ginseng was planted in beds shaded by lath slats, or under wire covered by fast-growing annual vines. But growers found it took seven years to produce roots large enough to market, and then the roots lacked the quality of those gathered in the wild. Garden plants were subject to a variety of wilts, blights, and rots, and a whole garden could be decimated in a week. But even though they were a gamble, ginseng gardens continued to appeal to many who wished to make an easy fortune.

However, the most money continued to be in gathering wild ginseng. Around 1922, someone wrote: "Grandma B. took out the back seat of her Model T and filled it with ginseng and sold the load for $1,100. They dried the roots on shelves behind the stove." As ginseng disappeared in more settled parts of the country, sang hunting in the Appalachians continued. Maurice Brooks wrote that it was one of the few crops that could be sold for cash with which to pay taxes or buy a new gun or hound dog. The sang hunter would go off into the mountains or woodlands with his special sanghoe made of rigid steel with a narrow blade. The average-sized wild roots weighed up to six ounces when dug, and an expert sanger could grub out two pounds in a day. As *they dried, usually from the cabin rafters, it took five pounds of fresh root for each pound of cured or marketable root.*

The conservate sanger only dug roots in the fall of the year and carefully replanted the seeds, or the rhizome extension called a "quill," or "bud." To keep ginseng from being completely killed out in an area, some sangers would carry seeds and plant them in other suitable locales. There were, however, those greedy individuals who gathered sang at any time of the year, and did not hesitate to rob a neighbor's patch. Sang hunters would try to find out where their competitors had success, and in turn would keep their own finds a secret. By 1913, Horace Kephart, in "Our Southern Highlands," wrote that ginseng had been exterminated in all but the wildest regions.

After the war in Korea ruined most original ginseng lands, the sale of ginseng roots reached a new peak, the price rising to $35.00 a pound for wild roots. Sangers scoured the country for roots and dealers made and lost fortunes on ginseng sales.

The price is still high, and while some ginseng is being brought to dealers from Illinois, Missouri, West Virginia, and Kentucky, the bulk now comes from North Carolina, Tennessee and Georgia.

Ginseng is slowly dying out. Since people first discovered that "sang hunting" could be a profitable hobby, they have been digging it more and more with less and less regard for its safety. Now, because of its scarcity and the increased demand for it, the price that dealers pay hunters for the dried roots has skyrocketed to $65.00 a pound! [2]

One early Latter-day Saint who remembered these familiar "sang hunts" was Henry William Bigler. Born in 1815 in Harrison County, West Virginia, he relates the following:

The month of August and forepart of September was the time to dig ginseng and snakeroot. They were articles the merchants readily exchanged goods for. Sang was found in the woods in the rich heads of hollows or in the most fertile parts, while snakeroot was found on thinner soil among the beech timber. Sang was easily discovered by its rich yellow leaves and red berries that grew on the stalks about a foot high.[2a]

At the heighth of this flourishing business in the early 1800s, an honest farmer of humble means investigated this lucrative venture with the prospect in mind of turning a dollar or two in the hopes of bettering his large family. The man was none other than Joseph Smith, Senior, first patriarch to the Church of Jesus Christ of Latter-day Saints, and father to the Mormon Prophet, Joseph Smith. His story is an interesting one and sheds some light upon the influence which herbal teas had upon the mind of his young boy, Joseph Junior. His wife, Lucy Mack Smith, recounts it as follows:

> *My husband, as before stated, followed merchandising for a short period in the town of Randolph. Soon after he commenced business in this place, he ascertained that crystalized ginseng root sold very high in China, being used as a remedy for the plague, which was then raging there.*
>
> *He therefore concluded to embark in a traffic of this article, and consequently made an investment of all the means which he commanded, in that way and manner which was necessary to carry on a business of this kind, viz, crystalizing and exporting the root. When he had obtained a quantity of the same, a merchant by the name of Stevens, of Royalton, offered him three thousand dollars for what he had, but my husband refused his offer, as it was only about two-thirds of its real value, and told the gentleman that he would rather venture shipping it himself.*
>
> *My husband, in a short time, went to the city of New York, with the view of shipping his ginseng, and finding a vessel in port which was soon to set sail, he made arrangements with the captain to this effect—that he was to sell the ginseng in China, and return the avails thereof to my husband, and this the captain bound himself to do, in a written obligation.*
>
> *Mr. Stevens, hearing that Mr. Smith was making arrangements to ship his ginseng, repaired immediately to New York, and, by taking some pains, he ascertained the vessel on board of which Mr. Smith had shipped his ginseng, and having some of the same article on hand himself, he made arrangements with the captain to take his also, and he was to send his son on board the vessel to take charge of it.*
>
> *It appears, from circumstances that afterward transpired, that the ginseng was taken to China, and sold there to*

good advantage, or at a high price, but not to much advantage to us, for we never received anything, except a small chest of teas of the avails arising from this adventure.

When the vessel returned, Stevens the younger also returned with it, and when my husband became apprised of his arrival, he went immediately to him and made inquiry respecting the success of the captain in selling his ginseng. Mr. Stevens told him quite a plausible tale, the particulars of which I have forgotten; but the amount of it was, that the sale had been a perfect failure, and the only thing which had been brought for Mr. Smith from China, was a small chest of tea, which chest had been delivered into his care, for my husband.

In a short time after this young Stevens hired a house of Major Mack, and employed eight or ten hands, and commenced the business of crystalizing ginseng. Soon after engaging in this business, when he had got fairly at work, my brother, Major Mack, went to see him, and, as it happened, he found him considerably intoxicated. When my brother came into his presence, he spoke to him thus, "Well, Mr. Stevens, you are doing a fine business; you will soon be ready for another trip to China." Then observed again, in a quite indifferent manner, "Oh, Mr. Stevens, how much did Brother Smith's adventure bring?" Being under the influence of liquor, he was not on his guard, and took my brother by the hand and led him to a trunk; then opening it, he observed, "There, sir, are the proceeds of Mr. Smith's ginseng!" exhibiting a large amount of silver and gold.

My brother was much astounded at this; however, he disguised his feelings, and conversed with him a short time upon different subjects, then returned home, and about ten o'clock the same night he started for Randolph, to see my husband.

When Mr. Stevens had overcome his intoxication, he began to reflect upon what he had done, and making some inquiry concerning my brother, he ascertained that he had gone to Randolph. Mr. Stevens, conjecturing his business—that he had gone to see my husband respecting the ginseng adventure—went immediately to his establishment, dismissed his hands, called his carriage, and fled with his cash for Canada, and I have never heard anything concerning him since.

My husband pursued him a while, but finding pursuit

vain, returned home much dispirited at the state of his affairs. He then went to work to overhaul his accounts, in order to see how he stood with the world; upon which he discovered that, in addition to the loss sustained by the China adventure, he had lost about two thousand dollars in bad debts. At the time he sent his venture to China he was owing eighteen hundred dollars in the city of Boston, for store goods, and he expected to discharge the debt at the return of the China expedition; but, having invested almost all his means in ginseng, the loss which he suffered in this article rendered it impossible for him to pay his debt with the property which remained in his hands. The principal dependence left him in the shape of property, was the farm at Tunbridge, upon which we were then living, having moved back to this place immediately after his venture was sent to China. This farm, which was worth about fifteen hundred dollars, my husband sold for eight hundred dollars, in order to make a speedy payment on the Boston debt; and, as I had not used the check of one thousand dollars which my brother and Mr. Mudget gave me, I added it to the eight hundred dollars obtained for the farm, and by this means the whole debt was liquidated. [3]

Thus, we can see that the tea business proved an utter and complete failure for Mr. Smith. However, from the facts on hand, we are able to learn this from the narrative just given:

(a) No mention is made in Mother Smith's account of her husband having to hire out labor to process the stuff as his partner, Mr. Stevens, had to do afterwards. This, then, apparently indicates that his own family participated in the venture together. Inasmuch as they were close and rather large in number, it would only seem logical to think that the man would use his own sons and daughters to help him in whatever capacity he needed them, in order to process the tea in crystalized form for export to China. Hence, his young son Joseph would have been employed somehow, too, thus bringing the youngster in contact with herbs. Who can but say that through his handling of the roots and such, it may not have evoked questions from his bright and inquisitive mind as to the Nature and purpose of the curious substance before him. Certainly, some discussion of it among family members would have had a slight bearing on his youthful and retentive memory, which would affect his judgment later on while in manhood.

(b) The "small chest of tea" given Father Smith, as a pecuniary reward for his large efforts of investment, obviously put the herb right into the Smith home. Though Mother Smith is silent upon its use thereafter, certainly it would be safe in assuming that something so treasured and highly valued as this commodity would surely find some purpose in their household, besides collecting dust or being discarded later on. So, from handling the herb and having it in their home, young Joseph Smith became intimately acquainted with one of Nature's finest healing properties: the ginseng plant.

Sir Edwin Arnold, the famous British writer and student of Eastern peoples, said of its medicinal values:

> *"According to the Chinamen, Ginseng is the best and most potent of cordials, of stimulants, of tonics, of stomachics, cardiacs, febrifuges, and above all, will best renovate and reinvigorate failing forces. It fills the heart with hilarity while its occasional use will, it is said, add a decade of years to the ordinary human life. Can all these millions of Orientals, all those many generations of men, who have boiled Ginseng in silver kettles and have praised heaven for its many benefits, have been totally deceived? Was the world ever quite mistaken when half of it believed in something never puffed, nowhere advertized, and not yet fallen to the fate of a Trust, a Combine or a Corner?"*[4]

When he was head of his own household some years later, the Prophet always felt to keep herb teas on hand. As early as 1833, we are furnished with evidence and proof of this statement:

> *I know persons who apostatized because they supposed they had reasons; for instance, a certain family, after having travelled a long journey, arrived in Kirtland, and the Prophet asked them to stop with him until they could find a place. Sister Emma, in the meantime, asked the old lady if she would have a cup of tea to refresh her after the fatigues of the journey...This whole family apostatized because they were invited to take a cup of tea...after the Word of Wisdom was given.*[5]

Now, it may here be asked, "Was the kind offer of the Prophet's wife going against the Word of Wisdom?" And again, we may query, "Is it against the Word of Wisdom to drink herb teas?" Finally, "Did the Prophet himself feel that tea was a part of the Word of Wisdom?"

We begin this short discussion by answering the last question first. Joel H. Johnson, who was intimately acquainted with Joseph Smith, said that on the Sabbath of July 1833, he heard the Prophet make this clear distinction about that beverage in question:

> *I understand that some of the people are excusing themselves in using tea...because the Lord only said 'hot drinks' in the revelation of the Word of Wisdom. Tea...(is) what the Lord meant when he said 'hot drinks.'*[6]

Now, the Lord had said in the Doctrine and Covenants: "And again, hot drinks *ARE NOT* for the body or belly."[7] Therefore, it would seem to be a sort of puzzlement at first in regards to what God had said upon the matter, and His servant, thereafter, detailing the specifics of what He had meant. But upon a more careful examination of the subject at large, one is able to see a consistent harmony between the two, and yet at the same time realizing that both *WERE NOT* against the contents, but rather the *DEGREE OF HEAT* to which they were served.

The Widstoes, John A. and Leah D., considered the most reputable authorities upon the Word of Wisdom and its broad interpretation in modern times, had this to say about the temperature of that liquid:

> *The Meaning of "Hot Drinks." When the Word of Wisdom was first promulagated in 1833, the question was at once asked: What is the meaning of "hot drinks"? Was it an injunction against consuming beverages so hot as to burn the tongue or mouth? That did not seem reasonable. Did it mean that the consumption of warm drinks should be reduced? That did not, even in that day, seem so unreasonable, for it was recognized that the stomach lining might be made unduly sensitive by frequent large ingestions of hot liquids. In fact, some clinical results of the modern day indicate that hot beverages, continuously used, predispose the stomach to certain serious disorders.*[8]

President Brigham Young, who was very near the Prophet, taught the people in the same manner:

> *This Word of Wisdom prohibits the use of hot drinks...I have heard it argued that tea [is] not mentioned therein; that is very true; but what were the people in the habit of taking as hot drinks when that revelation was given? Tea...We were not in the habit of drinking water very hot, but tea...the [beverage] in common use.*[9]

However, it may be well worth stressing at this juncture of things, that *certain kinds* of tea have always been understood to be *AGAINST* the Word of Wisdom. Such teas would include black tea, orange pekoe tea, and the commercial variety of related substances commonly found in today's supermarket. Famous name brands advertized by television and screen personalities are the ones in mention. The reason that such are *DEFINITELY AGAINST* the Word of Wisdom is because of what they contain. Again, we refer to the Widstoes for a definite clarity of this harmful element:

> *Tannic acid in tea to a large extent, is an astringent. It is found in oakbark and is the active substance in the tanning of leather. When tannic acid is taken into the body, its astringent Nature affects the lining and the contents of the stomach and intestines, tending to cause many serious disorders. A practical recognition of the injurious effect of tannic acid is the advice to steep tea quickly in hot water, so that the caffeine, which is very soluble, may go into solution, while the less soluble tannic acid in large part remains behind. Long continued steeping of tea leaves brings the tannic acid into a more complete solution and makes the resulting tea a more dangerous beverage.*[10]

But to show the reader that there is a distinct difference between the two, we refer to the published account in church history work, which leaves no doubt whatsoever, that herb tea IS NOT against the Word of Wisdom. The Prophet himself, being very ill at the time, had such nostrums of Nature, as what his condition required, faithfully administered unto him by his herbal physician, Dr. Levi Richards.

> *Monday, June 12, 1837. I was taken sick...*
>
> *Tuesday, 13.—My afflictions continued to increase and were very severe, insomuch that I was unable to raise my head from my pillow...*
>
> *Wednesday, 14.—I continued to grow worse and worse until my sufferings were excruciating...I found it expedient to call to my assistance those means which a kind Providence had provided for the restoration of the sick, in connection with the ordinances; and Dr. Levi Richards, at my request, administered to me HERBS...I began to amend in a short time.* [11]

However, the letter of the law seemed to prevail more among some of the orthodox in the Church then, than did the Spirit of it. We find Oliver Cowdery being brought up against the high council at Far West on certain charges of not keeping the Word of Wisdom. He was accused of drinking tea among other things. Oliver answered this charge by saying that he had drunk tea three times a day during that winter, but only on account of his poor and feeble health.[12] Due to the fact that his consumption of this beverage came under the herbal rather than something else, these particular accusations were dropped, seeing as how they were not sufficient grounds upon which to try him.

Yet a radical spirit of strict adherence to the letter caused some sanctimonious Saints in Kirtland to only drink cold water, and not even mention the word tea or suggest any benefits which might have been derived from the same.[13]

One of the principal men involved in this straightlaced attitude about the Word of Wisdom was Sidney Rigdon, a leading pillar in the Church at that time, and a member of the First Presidency, in fact. As one Mormon writer described him, he was "strict and rigid."[14] Perhaps this can account for the fact that for some time he did not partake of any herbal remedies, feeling that the teas which they constituted were against the revealed will of God.

Therefore, whenever he was sick, he would consult the services of a prominent medical physician to attend him, rather than an herbalist. A classic illustration of this may be found in the following:

> *Thursday, October 31, 1839—We tarried at Quincy to complete the necessary papers for our mission. Elder Rigdon was sick.*
>
> *Saturday, November 2—Continued our journey, and during the day put up with a friend on the bank of the Illinois river, so that Dr. Foster, who had accompanied us so far for that purpose, might administer medicine to Elder Rigdon again.*[15]

So that the reader may not be misled into thinking that Dr. Foster was an herbalist, like Dr. Levi Richards, it may do well to state he was an "M.D., a gentleman of great energy of character, late of Adams Co."[16] But, a few years later, Sidney had mended his ways somewhat, changed his opinion about such 'nonsense,' and became fully convinced that what Brother Joseph took for his ills was the right thing after all to do.

It was at the time of the Mormon expulsion from Missouri and their subsequent settlement in Commerce the following year (1839), that Joseph Smith remarked, "The Saints should use wisdom, and this is wisdom—if a cup of tea will stop a chill and fever, *USE IT*, but only to drive away the seizure." When the poor Saints were suffering by the hundreds from the ague fever and chill, he generously administered tea unto them and said it was wisdom to do so and check the ague.[17]

Being as closely connected to Joseph as he was, Elder Rigdon, undoubtedly, took this message to heart, for we find him immediately buying "1/2 lb. of tea at $1.25," from a local mercantile store set up by one of the brethren then. The date of this transaction was October 22, 1839, and his purchase must have brought some relief to him, for, thereafter, he frequented said establishment several times more for that unnamed tea to which he had now become converted.[18]

The extent to which herbal tea was applied in the Mormon diet of liquids may be readily seen from the following information:

> *Wednesday, September 18, 1839. Went to Burlington, Iowa Territory. Elders Young and Kimball left Sister Kimball and all her children sick, except little Heber; went thirteen miles on their journey towards England, and were left at Brother Osmun M. Duel's, who lived in a small cabin near the railway between Commerce and Warsaw. They were so feeble as to be unable to carry their trunks into the house without the assistance of Sister Duel, who received them kindly, prepared a bed for them to lie on, and MADE THEM A CUP OF TEA.*[19]

* * *

(Amos Davis Store Accounts)

August 15, 1839

Wm. Smith—peppermint tea		.25
castor oil		.50
(returned flask)		

October 9, 1839

O. Granger—2 lbs. butter	20	40
1/4 lbs. tea		3.5
1/4 lbs. salts		
1 doz. eggs		12.5

November 7, 1839

Ables (The Mormon Negro Convert, Elijah Abel)

Rum	31
Camphor	
Pine Bark	51.25

November 16, 1839			
H(yrum) Smith—	1 Box Lee's Nat. Herb Pills 25		
December 10, 1839			
Samuel Bent—	lb. Ginseng-Pepperment Tea	1.25	
V(inson) Knight—	1/2 lb. Tea	1.00	
E. Able—	1/4 lb. Tea		
January 1, 1840			
Markham—	1/4 lb. Tea 1.00	50	50
Kreymeyer—	1/4 lb. Tea	31k	31k
January 21, 1840			
N(ewel) Knight—	1/4 lb. Tea	25	100
	1 qt. molasses	25	
January 25, 1840			
Nelson Higgins—	1/4 lb. Tea	25	25
February 22, 1840			
Orson Hyde—	1 lb. Tea	125	125
Able cr(edit)	4 lb. Tea	50	
L(evi) Jackman—	Pencil	6 2/3	56 2/3
March 2, 1840			
Wm. Jackson—	8 doz. eggs	124	100
	2 lbs. sugar	124	25
	1/4 " Tea	125	31 1/4
March 18, 1840			
Squire Bosworth—	1/4 lbs. Tea	37 1/4	
	1/4 lbs. spice		
	1 Tea Pot	62 1/4	62 1/420

And, of course, such frequent usage of these herbal means always followed in the wake of a remark or two Joseph might have happened to make on the occasions in which he did these things.

His attitude relative to the consumption of herbal beverages is best summed up by these enlightening remarks of a mormon researcher in modern times:

> *Joseph's approach to the Word of Wisdom, when viewed in historical perspective, seems sensible and rational. In the later 1830s, the Kirtland Stake had dissolved due to apostasy; the Missouri Saints were being driven from the state with accompanying hardships, and Joseph himself was imprisoned. At a time when the Church was struggling for more existence, it would seem small and petty to quibble about a drink of tea... Emphasis on a rigid interpretation of a health code during such a period of turmoil would seem ill-timed and inappropriate. Moreover, there is some evidence that Joseph sought to avoid needless dissension among the Saints by urging moderation and charity.*[21]

Thus, we can see from a sympathetic approach by way of Spirit, rather than a tyrannical resolve by way of letter, the Prophet was able to receive the wonderful benefits and derive the excellent blessings contained in the use of herbal teas, as well as to enjoin his followers in the same practice likewise.

The more faithful portion of the Church, who adopted their leader's wise actions, received a restoration of full and complete health when they heeded the same:

> *Saturday, 2, — This morning I found myself quite unwell with a threatening of the horrible ague and when I arose I found Brother Holme's folks doctoring one of his sons for the same complaint. They said he had been sick most of the night and they wanted I should take some also. But I told them if I did take their medicine, I shouldn't be able to go with Brother R.. Therefore, I went into the woods and told my Heavenly Father if it was his will I should go and wanted that He should rebuke the disorder of my body. I waited until half past 10 and Brother R. did not come. I began to think it was not the Will of God for us to go, for my disease grew worse. I went to bed and BEGAN TO TAKE SOME WARM HERB DRINK and got to sweating considerable freely; and then took one of Dr. Thompson's emetick (a natural laxative). The Lord BLESSED IT, and I began to be better. While I was under the operation of this, Brother R. came and he said he was not much surprised for his wife told him when he was starting, she did not think he would go any farther than Brother H's and home again. We soon returned. When the emetick had done operating, I felt much better than I had for some time*

before.[22]

In the month of February, 1841, on the 15th, Joseph Smith made this small notation in his journal:

> *I spoke at great length...that roots and herbs can be found to effect all necessary purposes (of healing).*[23]

And just a year previous to this, we find a small festivity got up among some of the brethren in England:

> *Sunday, May 17—Elders Young, Woodruff, and Richards held conference with the Saints at Gadfield Elm Chapel.*
>
> *Monday, May 18—The above Elders met the brethren at Elder Kingston's where they had a tea party, praying, singing, confirming, ordaining, and about twenty were baptized.*[24]

Apparently, herb drink was good enough to use in so solemn a manner of spiritual celebration.

During the Nauvoo period, Brigham Young took quite a liking to tea, and concocted a formula of herbal blend which seemed rather satisfying and popular among the Saints then:

> *The Mormons also used Brigham Young's favorite drink, Composition Tea, made from herbs and spices. The prescription reads: "4 ounces each of ground bayberry, poplar bark and hemlock; 2 ounces each of ground ginger, cloves and cinnamon; 1 ounce of cayenne pepper." Directions: "Take a small bit on a spoon, put in a cup of hot water, with plenty of sugar and cream."*[25]

After the beloved Prophet's unfortunate martyrdom, his successor, President Young, maintained the same type of philosophy in regards to these natural beverages:

> *...of a truth...where a person is diseased, say, for instance, with canker, there is no better medicine than green tea, and where it is thus used, it should be drank sparingly.*[26]

Again, like Joseph, recommending herbal tea for sickness, but to be used with wisdom and discretion.

Brigham further elaborated upon the general theme of drinking tea as espoused in the revelation given that matter:

> *The Word of Wisdom is one thing, and ignorance, superstition, or bigotry is another. I wish people to come to an understanding with regard to the Word of Wisdom. For illustration, I will refer to a certain brother who was in the church once, and President of the Elder's Quorum in Nauvoo. While living at that place there was a great deal of sickness among the people, and he was sometimes called in to lay hands on the sick, but if he had the least doubt about their drinking tea, if he even saw a teapot, he would refuse. I recollect he went into a house where a woman was sick, who wanted him to lay hands on her; he saw a teapot in the corner containing catnip tea, but without stopping to inquire he left the house, exclaiming against her and her practices.*
>
> *...Do not throw these things away, and say they must never be used; they are good to be used with judgment, prudence and discretion.*[27]

It would do well for some in our time to carefully examine what President Young has said, and review themselves and their prejudiced attitudes towards others in the light of these inspired words from a living oracle of God.

The Saints continued to use such things as they crossed the Plains. Faced with the uncertainties of sickness and disease, they sought to stave off death by employing the practical means they knew about, which were at their constant disposal. However, again the bigotry of some narrow-minded Latter-day Saints, who would "strain at a gnat, to swallow a camel," crept into an otherwise perfectly acceptable practice in the sight of God, and turned such moments of natural reliance into bitter and painful experiences, long to be remembered thereafter:

> *One night when we came into camp, it was after dark and had been raining very, very hard through the day and there was no wood to be got and Mother was very sick. We thought she was going to die and we had gathered a few sunflower stalks and wet buffalo chips and had just got a little fire started, when all hands were ordered to attend prayers, and because we did not go to prayers, Daniel Taylor came and kicked our fire all out and spilled the water that we were trying to get warm to MAKE A LITTLE TEA for Mother. I then told him if I ever got to be a man [Heber was 13 at the time of this incident] I would whip him if it was the last thing I ever did on this earth. Father had gone to attend prayers and that was the reason he took advantage of*

us. Well, this is about the way we had to get along and pass through the same every day.[27]

Tea drinking was once considered a social grace within the Church:

Parley P. Pratt went to Hamilton. He had no money. He entered a forest to pray for money, to go to Toronto. After pouring his soul forth in prayer, he returned to the city. A stranger accosted him on the street; asked his name and where he was going. This man also asked Parley if he did not want some money; and gave him $10.00, together with a letter of introduction to Mr. John Taylor of Toronto. Parley thanked this gentleman very kindly, and departed for Toronto, where he arrived the same evening. Mrs. John Taylor received him kindly, and went for her husband, who was at his mechanic shop near by. Parley told them his errand; but did not receive much encouragement from Mr. Taylor. Parley TOOK TEA with them, and sought lodging at a public house.[28]

However, the factors of hardship and difficulty soon changed all of that and what had been "good etiquette" soon became a necessary predicate:

[January 3, 1856] Mary Gustin called in on her return from the city giving me a verbal message from Mr. Heywood that if my children were taken with the measles to give them saffron tea or bran water.

February 22—Nearly was taken sick in the morning, complained of a sore mouth, headache, had several diarrhea passages during the day and threw up phlegm twice or thrice, breath smelled very bad of canker. Doctored at once for the canker and also gave him some SAFFRON AND SAGE TEA. Next day continued very sick and showed some rash, fever high. Towards night I bathed him all over with saleratus water and the rash or measles came out very full, so I continued to give him SAFFRON TEA AND SAGE. He was very sick but took a turn on Tuesday 26th for the better. [30]

Herbal medicine, in the form of warm, mild drinks, was also administered in cases of difficult child-labor:

In the summer of 1884, in Kane County, in Orderville,

UT., I was called to a young lady with her first child. She had been in labor 2 or 3 days and was give up by the midwives for a surgeon who they wanted to send for right off; saying she was malformed and never could be delivered only by taking a bit at a time. They were much opposed to me and my medicine, but by the influence of friends they said I might try what I could do. I gave her the same course with the same kind of medicines as in other cases and in due time the child came.

Composition powder: Thompson's Bayberry bark 2 lbs.; hemlock bark 1 lb.; ginger root 1 lb.; cayenne pepper 2 ozs.; cloves 2 ozs.; all finely pulverized and well mixed. Dose: one half of a teaspoon and a spoonful of sugar, put them into a tea cup and pour it half full of boiling water; let it stand a few minutes. Fill the cup with milk, and drink freely. If no milk is to be obtained, fill up the cup with hot water.

This, in the first stages and less violent attacks of the disease, is a valuable medicine, and may be safely employed in all cases. It is good to relax pain in the stomach and bowels and to remove all obstructions caused by cold. A few doses, the patient being in bed with a steaming stone at the feet, or having soaked the feet fifteen or twenty minutes in hot water, drinking freely of the tea at the same time, will cure a bad cold, and often throw off the disease in its first stages.[31]

Early pioneer herbalists, such as Dr. John L. Dunyon, who happened to be President Brigham Young's medical advisor and practicing physician as well as with other leading families in the Church, had a combination of natural ingredients which were intended to rejuvenate the system of a person, thereby increasing one's longevity. He called it the Elixir of Life, and its formula went this way:

1 lb. gum myrrh, 1/2 lb. aloes, 1/4 lb. saffron, 1/2 lb. hops, 1/2 lb. rhubarb, 1/2 lb. camomile, 2 oz. cayenne, 4 oz. cinnamon, 4 oz. cloves, 1 lb. anise seed. Add water to cover well, strain, boil and add water so that there will be 5 to 6 gallons in all. Take lb. each of the following, either poplar, boneset, jimson or balmory. Boil in water, strain and boil down so as to make in all 8 gallons, then add sugar, boil it with the bitter decoction and skim, then add it to the former mixture, flavor with the essence of wintergreen and bottle. Dose: 1 ths. six times a day.[32]

Herbal doctors had definite purposes for certain kinds of native plants:

My grandfather, Henry Hughes, was a doctor of herbs. At the annual fair held at Logan City, Cache County in September, 1880, he was awarded a diploma for the best collection of medicinal plants by the Cache County Agricultural and Manufacturing Society. He went among the sick taking various herbs with him which he STEEPED INTO A TEA... My Grandmother went with him as a nurse. They received very little remuneration for their services and gave it willingly to all in need.

Among the medicine used by my grandparents were:

Wild sage simmered in water and strained with a little whiskey to preserve it. It was used as a tonic and also for hot packs in cases of bruises and abscesses. Tame Sage STEEPED SLOWLY FOR A TEA is used for upset stomach; also when mashed up in a tsp. of olive oil was used for worms. Verbine tea was used to induce perspiration.

Brookline tea, for the blood was taken in the spring. Wormwood in large amounts of water, simmered down to a small amount, and some brandy added was considered a sure cure for Mountain Fever. Rabbit Brush and Tea Weed was used for rheumatism. Marshmallow Weed was used for poultices and hot packs in cases of infection.

Clover Blossom tea was used to build up the blood. Elm Bark combined with yeast was used as a poultice for ulcers when there was a tendency to gangrene; also used as an antiseptic. Peach Tree Leaves SIMMERED IN WATER was used as a sedative, controls nausea and vomiting.[33]

Others, besides the prophets, had sensible remedies for certain ills:

Emma Helene (Lena) Colton Davis sold to the people of Minersville and surrounding communities, a canker medicine said to be exceptionally good: 2 lbs. lump borax, 2 tbs. alum, 1 tbs. copperas. Burn each separately on an iron griddle. Steep one handful of garden sage in 14 qts. boiling water, strain and add the above ingredients, plus tsp. nutmeg. Boil about 10 min. or until dissolved. Set aside overnight. In the morning pour off clear liquid and add 14 cups of honey, 4 sugar and 2 tsp. golden seal to the liquid. Boil 10 min., strain through clean cloth, then heat again. After it has cooled a little while, bottle. Use for sore throats and all mouth and throat irritations.[34]

Brigham did not hesitate to recommend specific herbs to overcome certain kinds of bad habits:

I wish to ask those brethren who are in the habit of using tobacco, won't you leave it alone and try lobelia, and see if you can become attached to it?[35]

In regards to illness, the Prophet of God carried on in the same tradition which his dear friend, Joseph Smith had done. He gave some sound medical advice for parents to follow when their youngsters are not feeling well. Those who are wise and intelligent will put their trust in a man of God rather than in antibiotics or innoculations:

Doctors and their medicines I regard as a deadly bane to any community. Give your children, when sick, A LITTLE SIMPLE HERB DRINK; and if they have eaten too much let them go without food until their stomachs are cleansed and purified, and have faith in the name of Jesus and in the ordinances of his Church, and they will live. THAT IS MY FAITH with regard to this thing.[35a]

One faithful Latter-day Saint who placed such a confidence in the prophets rather than in the doctors, related this miraculous circumstance involving the use of herb tea in times of sickness:

My mother had dropsy. She became so swollen that it was impossible for her to lie down to sleep. She had been administered to many times. One day when she had been very bad my father and his brother, Uncle David Johnson, administered to her. From that time on she began to get better, until she was completely well. One day a stranger came walking down the road leading a donkey. He asked for water for the animal. As the animal drank he and Father stood there talking. Father told him his wife was very sick, and that there wasn't a doctor within a hundred miles. The stranger listened and seemed very much concerned. He asked several questions about her and then said, "You follow that trail that I just came over and about a quarter of a mile back you will find a bed of herbs with little yellow flowers on it. Gather it, steep it, and GIVE HER THE TEA. I am sure it will help her." Father thanked him kindly. He lost no time in getting the herbs and MAKING THE TEA.

One night my daughter, Ellen, had such a bad sore throat. I think it was what we would call Quincy now. Her throat was swollen so badly it was hard for her to breathe. There were no doctors. My husband was away from home and I was all alone. I had tried everything I knew. I went into another room and earnestly prayed for help. A voice spoke to me and told me what to do. I prepared the poultice and put it on her throat. She soon received relief and went to sleep. I used this same remedy many times, and it always worked. [35b]

Other servants of the Most High, who bore a swift and vivid witness to the truthfulness of Brigham's remarks were President George A. Smith and President Wilford Woodruff. Of the two, the former had this to say:

I do not have it now; I do not get tea for people, unless they pretend to be sick, then I tell my folks to make them a tin cup full of good, strong catnip tea. That is a rule I have prescribed.[36]

And the latter urged the Latter-day Saints to "lay aside whiskey, tobacco, TEA, and coffee, and use none of them unless it be AS A MEDICINE![37]

Despite the change in attitudes and policies, Joseph Smith's original suggestion to use herb teas in times of poor health has somehow managed to weather the sophistry of twentieth-century philosophy and survive amid the clamor of the "new theology" sweeping the nation these days. One man who kept it alive, in a semi-private sense at least, was President Anthony W. Ivins, of the Church's First Presidency. A missionary assigned to Mexico at the turn of the century briefly relates a visit this high church official made to that area, and reports a synopsis of what was said by him then:

Ozumba, Mexico. 23 Monday, May, 1904

This morning there was a meeting for the Elders in which Apostle Woodruff and Pres. Ivins gave us some pointed instructions... Pres. Ivins told us to carry along with us some simple remedies (of herbs) which would be useful in guarding prevalent ills.[38]

Another prominent General Authority within recent times, Apostle John A. Widstoe, extolled the virtues of such natural drinks in these beautiful words:

> *Infusions of herbs or herb teas are used in many countries of Europe. In France one may be served "infusion" of dried leaves of the verbena, mint and many herbs or the flowers of camomile, orange, or linden trees, much more frequently than the real China or India tea. A consequent improvement in health may definitely be noticed. They act as a tonic to the system and PROVE VERY BENEFICIAL. Everyone remembers the hop tea, dandelion or camomile teas of grandmother's day which were given as the annual spring tonic. There are many times when WARM (not too hot) HERB DRINKS ARE indicated and DESIRABLE.*[39]

His good wife shared similar views:

> *Herbs, teas or infusions may also be curative and medicinal as well as tonic in their effects.One might do well to use occasionally the herb drinks of the pioneers—catnip, camomile, and other "teas" which help to tone up the system as well as to relieve the monotony of diet.*[39a]

However, nothing comes quite so near these few simple words, expressed by one Lorenzo Brown, who was a veteran in the Utah War campaign and a member of the Mormon Militia which went against Albert Sidney Johnston's army in 1857:

> *September 30th. Had rations of beef, onions and tea, and after breakfast A GOOD CUP OF NICE HERB TEA. Felt quite well after that.*[40]

Basically speaking, it is this last description which fits so well the use of natural beverages within our eating economy. To use Lorenzo Brown's own words, they are *GOOD* for our system, *NICE* and pleasant to the senses, and make one feel *QUITE WELL* after their consumption.

It is a remarkable coincidence of history to relate that the Mormons were not the only ones with a revealed Word of Wisdom. Scarcely eight years after our historic revelation was given, the Shaker societies of upper New England received a similar correspondence from a supernatural source. As recorded in an old Shaker diary of December 16, 1841: "...Elder Grove had a communication given at New Lebanon concerning *TEA*, Swine, Meat, *all kinds of strong drink*, and coffee."[41] And what is even more incredible than this is that they were some of the principal characters behind the preparation and marketing of medicinal herbs and roots, which later spread to other segments of American society and were quickly adopted by the enterprising and business-minded. Other contributions which they bequeathed to this nation were: (a) they were the first to dry sweet corn for food; (b) the first to start the broom business in America; (c) the first to manufacture a buzz saw; and (d) the first to manufacture cut nails and metallic pens.[42] But it is to the establishment of the herb business on a large scale for which we are indebted to them the most. Though their peculiar type of society is no longer in existence anymore, yet the treasures in Mother Nature's magnificent pharmacy, which they so thoughtfully tapped and put to public use, shall always be remembered by those who enjoy such things with the fondest of care.

These old pioneer remedies are referred to in one of the D.U.P. lessons of the past which identifies plants used by the early settlers and gives a brief description of their practical use in various liquids of considerable worth:

> *Infusions: Compound Infusion of Geranium: take geranium root, sweet bugle leaves, golden seal root, witch-hazel bark, each, in coarse powder, one ounce; boiling water, four pints. Mix and allow to stand in covered vessel, two hours, applying gentle heat; then strain. Two drams of alum may or may not be added. Used in chronic diarrhea and dysentry, in one or two tablespoonful doses, every two or three hours. Also used as a gargle in ulcerations of the mouth and throat.*
>
> *Compound Infusion of Trailing Arbutus: Take a "queen of the meadow" root, dwarf elder bark, marshmallow root, and trailing arbutus each, coarsely bruised half an ounce, add to them one pint of boiling water, and one pint of Holland gin and steep by the fire four hours, in a closely covered vessel. Strain, and sweeten with honey. Excellent for gravel, suppression of urine, scalding of urine, and various other disorders of the urinary organs. Dose, from an ounce to a wineglassful, with more or less frequency, according to the urgency of the case.*
>
> *Hedge Mustard: Stimulus to the stomach and to relieve coughing. Also used in the form of an infusion (tea) to clean ulcers and wounds. Boil an ounce of seeds, or a quantity of leaves in a quart of water and wash sore parts twice a day.*
>
> *Hedge Nettle: Made into a tea and drank freely is excel-*

lent for hemorrhages of the lungs and stomach. In doses of one-half wineglassful four times a day, it relieves neuralgia. A poultice of the leaves also relieves neuralgic pains and aids in the cure of wounds. Used at times as a tea to promote menstruation and kill worms.

Asparagus: Used as a table dish stimulates the kidneys. In the form of a tea drunk at three or four hour intervals, it promotes the flow of urine.

Red Pepper: The pioneers used this as a gargle for scarlet fever. It was prepared by taking one-half teaspoonful of the pepper and one tablespoonful of table salt to a pint of boiling water. Thoroughly mix and strain and then add about a half teacupful of vinegar. Used frequently as a throat gargle. Give internally one-half teaspoonful every hour to a child, doubling the amount for adults. Red Pepper is also recommended as a cure for grippe, in the form of tea of the pods or the ground pepper. One tsp. to a half pint of water. Place a teaspoonful of the tea in a glass of hot water and drink slowly every three or four hours. In confinement, in hemorrhage cases, it should be taken cold. Taken hot it was used to begin labor.

Blue Flag Root: Wash and clean. Pound it, add a little water, and strain out the milky juice. Add sufficient red pepper to make it a little hot to the taste. This ia an excellent remedy for dyspepsia. Dose one Tbs. three times daily. Benefits the action of the liver and the pepper also stimulates the stomach.

Barks: Barks should be gathered as soon as they will peel easily in the spring. Leaves and herbs should be collected just before they begin to fade in the autumn. Flowers, when they first begin to blossom. Seeds, just before they are ripe. Roots may be dug at any time, thoroughly washed, cleaned and dried.

American Poplar is a good tonic and is a good remedy for chronic rheumatism, dyspepsia and general debility. Use only the inner part, dried and powdered.

Old Bark may be given with advantage in fever and ague, diarrhea and bleeding of the lungs. It is also good as an external application. The acorns, when roasted, are believed to be a remedy for scrofula and other skin diseases. A strong tea of the bark has also been recommended as a wash for old sores and foul ulcers. A poultice made of powdered bark will relieve pain, and is also considered a good remedy for sores and ulcers. Dose: Make a tea of the bark and take in such quantities as may be deemed necessary.

Peak Bark is a sedative and will control nausea and vomiting. It also possesses mild tonic properties. Dose: Make a strong tea of the bark and drink a wineglassful three times a day.

Crab Apple Bark has been known to cure chronic rheumatism. The bark is powdered then put into a sufficient amount of whiskey to make a strong tonic. Take a wineglassful three times daily until a gallon is consumed.[43]

The general virtues in the above-mentioned herbs speak forth for themselves in this lesson message.

Thus, it would seem from what we have learned that the use of herbal tea was quite prolific in the Mormon diet and one of the main characteristics prevalent in their drinking habits. Such a course seems to have come about as a direct result of what their leaders taught and preached, and what ordinary common sense dictated to them as wisdom.

So, to reiterate the statements of the Prophets, we again quote Joseph Smith: "If a cup of tea will stop a chill and fever, *USE IT*; but only to drive away the seizure." And follow with an identical statement from his successor, President Brigham Young: "Doctors and their medicines I regard as a deadly bane to any community. Give your children, when sick, *A LITTLE SIMPLE HERB DRINK...*"

Now, Brigham Young believed in the Prophet, for he viewed Joseph Smith as the greatest living oracle to have graced the nineteenth century. He regarded Joseph's words as the mind and will of God himself. And believing so sincerely in this great man's teachings, he devoutly practiced what his leader had said with the utmost of zeal. After the death of Brigham Young, Elder George Q. Cannon, a member of the First Presidency of the Church, under the reign of John Taylor, made some appropriate remarks to the Latter-day Saints, in the new Tabernacle on Temple Square. It has been ninety-nine years since those eventful words have been uttered, yet their truthfulness continues to live on right into the twentieth century. It would be well for every Latter-day Saint to consider these things and examine them with the greatest of scrutiny and weigh them in the most careful manner of thought possible. For in these words is contained the life, health, and well being of every individual concerned, in relation to virtues, actions, and *EVEN THE USE OF HERBAL TEA* in our daily diet:

> *...we should...seek to have the spirit that animated him [Brigham Young], and to follow him as he followed Joseph, as he honored Joseph, as he revered Joseph, as he upheld Joseph, as he maintained Joseph, TOUCHING DOCTRINE AND COUNSEL, so that it appears to me if we are animated by the Spirit of God we will honor him and follow in his footsteps, as he followed Joseph, and as Joseph followed Christ.*[43a]

In conclusion then, we know how Brother Joseph advised us in regards to plant drink of natural origin. We also are acquainted with what Brother Young said upon the subject. Their words are before us; we cannot refute them. We can only choose to obey or disobey their wise counsel and sensible admonitions. If we have a testimony of Joseph Smith, it will be caused by that *SAME SPIRIT* which animated him. And, if it is in us also, the words and thoughts of Joseph Smith shall live in our lives forever as practiced deeds of daily use. It can be no other way.

NOTES

1. A. R. Harding, *Ginseng And Other Medicinal Plants;* Columbus, Ohio, 1936; pp. 39—40.

2. Eliot Wigginton, *Foxfire 3*; New York, 1975; pp. 245—249.

2a. *Journal of Henry William Bigler*, Church Historian's Office, Salt Lake.

3. Lucy Mack Smith, *Joseph Smith and His Progenitors*; Lamoni, Iowa, 1912; pp. 43-47.

4. Harding, *op. cit.*, p. 50.

5. *Journal of Discourses* 2:214. Hereafter, cited as *JD.*

6. Joel H. Johnson, *A Voice From The Mountains*; p. 12.

7. *Doctrine & Covenants* 89:9. Hereafter, cited as *D & C.*

8. John A. and Leah D. Widstoe, *The Word of Wisdom—A Modern Interpretation*; Salt Lake City, 1937; p.85.

9. *JD* 13:277.

10. Widstoes, *op. cit.*, pp. 91—92.

11. *Documentary History of the Church* 11:493. Here after cited as *DHC.*

12. *The Far West Record.* January 26, 1838; Church Historian's Office, Salt Lake City.

13. W.W. Phelps, in a letter written to his wife, commenting upon the strictness with which the Kirtland Saints lived the revelation (Word of Wisdom). *Journal History,* May 26, 1835; Church Library, Salt Lake City.

14. Paul H. Petersen, *An Historical Analysis Of The Word of Wisdom*; Master's thesis, August, 1972; p. 24; Harold B. Lee Library, Brigham Young University, Provo, Utah.

15. *DEC* 4:19

16. *Times & Seasons* 2:275.

17. Missionary Journal of Arnold Auer Reiser, October 4, 1899; Harold B. Lee Library, Brigham Young University, Provo, Utah.

18. Amos David Account Book (August 15, 1839 to October 15, 1842); Western Americana section, Marriott Library, University of Utah, Salt Lake City.

19. *DHC* 4:9—10.

20. Amos Davis, op. cit.

21. Petersen, op. cit., pp. 39-40.

22. Evan Melbourne Greene's Journal (January 15, 1833—April 1, 1835), Vol. I; Church Historian's Office, Salt Lake City.

23. The Journals Of Joseph Smith, Junior; Church Historian's Office, Salt Lake City. Under date of February 15, 1841. See also Petersen's thesis, *op. cit.*, p. 31.

24. *DEC* 4:131.

25. The Keokuk, Iowa, *Daily Gate City*, May 8, 1962. As reprinted by the *Missouri Historical Society Bulletin*. April, 1963, p. 299.

26. *JD* 12:403.

27. Autobiography of Heber Robert McBride, p. 16; Special Collections Dept., Harold B. Lee Library, BYU, Provo, Utah.

28. Dr. Daniel B. Hill, Richards, *Hill Family History*; Salt Lake, February, 1927; p. 13.

29. predicate—n. 1. *Logic.* That which is affirmed or denied of a subject. In these propositions, "Paper is white," "Ink is not white," *whiteness* is the *predicate* affirmed of paper and denied of ink. (*Webster's New International Dictionary of the English Language)*, Second Ed., Unabridged, Springfield, p. 1946.

30. Kate B. Carter, "And They Were Healed"; DUP Lesson For October, 1957; p. 72.

31. *Ibid.*, pp. 89—90.

32. *Ibid.*, p. 96.

33. *Ibid.*, pp. 103—104.

34. *JD* 13:275—276.

35. *JD* 13

35a. *JD* 14:109.

35b. "The Story of Phoebe E. Johnson"; Roberta Clayton Manuscripts Collection, Bx 3, fd. #147; Harold B. Lee Library, BYU.

36. *JD* 16:238.

37. *JD* 11:370.

38. Journal of S. Marsena Foster, Book One; Western Americana section, Marriott Library, University of Utah, Salt Lake City.

39. Widstoe, *op. cit.*, p. 225.

39a. Leah D. Widstoe, *How To Be Well;* Missouri, 1943; p. 411.

40. Lorenzo Brown Journal, under date mentioned in main context; Harold B. Lee Library, Special Collections, BYU, Provo, Utah.

41. E. Cecil McGavin, *The Historical Background of the Doctrine and Covenants*; Salt Lake City,1949; p. 164.

42. *Ibid.*, p. 165.

43. DUP Lesson For October, 1957, pp. 119—120.

43a. *JD* 19:233.

CHAPTER TWO

EAT YOUR GREENS

(Vegetables in the Mormon Diet)

Anybody who is acquainted with children knows how much the average youngster hates his greens with a passion. For it seems that such condiments as these are not always relished by the juvenile set as much as the junk foods of hamburgers, hot dogs, soda pop, and candies and sweets. Yet what they nor their parents may be aware of, is simply that the inclusion of these necessary vitals in one's daily fare happens to be more than just good nutrition. As a matter of fact, the Bible says *IT IS A COMMANDMENT* to eat these things.

In Genesis, the Lord gave Adam a specific instruction: "...thou shalt eat the herb of the field."[1] And by way of interpretation, reliable lexicographers define vegetable as "a plant; specif., in common use a *HERB*aceous plant cultivated for food, as the cabbage, turnip, potato, etc.; also, the edible part or parts of such plants."[2] And Leah D. Widstoe, wife of Apostle John A. Widstoe, gave her own meaning to the word "greens": "This term includes those plants whose leaves are used for vegetables—beet, rutabaga, and turnip tops, young dandelion leaves, chicory, outside lettuce leaves, escarole, Swiss chard, kale and spinach."[3] Thus, we can see that the law of health which the Almighty set down for Adam to follow included *vegetables* (*HERB*aceous plants) and *greens* (leafy vegetables).

Being an obedient servant by Nature, Adam sought to keep this law and thereby live according to the way which God had revealed to him. For his faithfulness and diligence in such a matter, God blessed his body, and according to Apostle Orson Pratt, "Adam and Eve ate *FRUITS AND VEGETABLES*, not animal flesh."[4]

In fact, so fine a physique did he have that the following description of his great strength and incredible speed was established by Joseph Smith:

St. George, April 16 (1182)—Father Jno. L. Lytle gave a very interesting account of his early experiences in the church, his travels with the Prophet Joseph and of his telling them how Father Adam chased the game, outstripped them, and caught them, and his knee was never brought to the ground, SO GREAT WAS HIS STRENGTH...[5]

Imagine, a man of his dynamic energy alive today! Why, not even the fictionalized accounts of a Six Million Dollar Man or a Superman could so accurately portray the human machine within the bounds of veracity and believability.

It is also an interesting thing worthy of record that Jacob of old, likewise, had a diet which consisted of much of the same things as Father Adam's did. We learn of this from the Good Book:

And the boys grew; and Esau was a cunning hunter, a man of the field; and Jacob was a plain man, dwelling in tents.

And Isaac loved Esau, because he did EAT OF HIS VENISON, but Rebekah loved Jacob.

And Jacob sod pottage; and Esau came from the field, and he was faint;...

Then Jacob gave Esau bread and pottage OF LENTILS.[6]

We are, therefore, able to see from a certain dish what type of food Jacob loved the most: namely, *LENTILS*, which are nothing more than good, old fashioned vegetables belonging to the pea family. And, it may here be asked, "Just what benefits did he derive from this type of eating?" The answer is a very logical one: *STRENGTH*, and lots of it. This can be proven from the Biblical account furnished us of his wrestling with an Angel all night long until the break of dawn.[7] For here is positive and absolute proof, that *A CONSISTENT DIET OF GREENS* (lentils) *GIVES ONE GREAT STRENGTH AND LONGEVITY*! Patriarch Jacob lived a total of one hundred and forty-seven years.[8] Not bad for that time, considering that the age of man had sharply decreased *AFTER* the Flood.

But the Bible is not through with commenting upon this type of food. Later on, we find in Proverbs 15:17: "Better is a dinner of herbs...than an ox...." Again, stressing the point of a natural meal over a heavy meat dinner. However, to the Latter-day Saints, God has been most specific:

And again, verily I say unto you, all wholesome herbs God hath ordained for the constitution, Nature and use of man.[9]

How much clearer could He be than this? And yet, so many of our generation today seem to flagrantly ignore the wisdom of Jehovah and flaunt His laws openly by their careless diet and neglectful eating habits. President Brigham Young foresaw this condition in modern times and remarked upon the same in the following appropriate manner:

...Where is the iron constitution, the marrow in the bone, the power in the loins, and the strength in the sinew and muscle of which the ancient fathers could boast? These have, in a great measure PASSED AWAY; they have decayed from generation to generation, until CONSTITUTIONAL WEAKNESS AND EFFEMINACY ARE BEQUEATHED TO US THROUGH THE IRREGULARITIES AND SINS OF OUR FATHERS! THE HEALTH and power and beauty THAT ONCE ADORNED the noble form of MAN MUST BE RESTORED TO OUR RACE; and God designs that we shall engage in this great work of restoration. Then let us not trifle with our mission, by indulging in the use of injurious substances. These lay the foundation of disease and death in the systems of men, and the same are committed to their children, and another generation of feeble human beings is introduced into the world. Such children have insufficient bone, sinew, muscle, and constitution, and are of little use to themselves, or to their fellow creatures; they are not prepared for life, but for the grave; not to live five, six, eight, and nine hundred years, but to appear for a moment, as it were, and pass away. Now, when a person is fifty years of age he or she is considered an old man or an old woman; they begin to feel decrepit, and think they must feel old, appear old, and begin to die. Premature death is in the marrow of their bones, the seeds of early dissolution are sown in their bodies, they feel old at fifty, sixty, and seventy years, when they should feel like boys of fifteen, sixteen, and seventeen. Instead of feeling decrepit at those years they should feel full of strength, vigor, and life, having attained to early maturity, prepared now to enter upon the duties of a long future life, and when two hundred years have been attained, they should then feel more vigorous than the healthiest of men do in this age at forty and fifty years. [10]

It seems rather strange, but the early Latter-day Saints enjoyed the benefits of natural greens more often than domestic produce when they were uprooted from their homes and forced to leave their properties.

The efficacy of such a truth may be seen in a statement made by Mosiah L. Hancock, relative to the early settlement of Nauvoo:

> *At times we children were so hungry and sick that it seemed we were destined to starve to death.... As hard as our lot was, we never quarrelled. Sometimes when our parents were sick and could not cook GREENS, we ate them raw. I have pulled up GRASS and ate it; also basswood buds and elmbark.*[11]

Furthermore, proof that the newcomers to Commerce (later renamed Nauvoo) did not have the time nor the means to grow their own vegetables may be readily seen in the account book of one Amos Davis, who kept a mercantile store there from August 15, 1839 until October 11, 1842. His ledger begins out with an occasional mention of "rice & onions to Saml. Smith" for 75 cents and 59 cents respectively. This transaction was completed and made September 7 of that first year. On October 4, Edward Farley bought "1 bushel onions" for 75 cents. November 16 a J.S. Miles purchased "Burkill Beens" for 50 cents. Actually, it was not until the Spring of 1840 that such interesting items as "1 bushel corn, Joshua Smith" for 46 cents first made their appearance. Thereafter, such entries as that of a Major Russell became rather common:

1 bushell potatoes	3 1/2
1/2 bushell turnups	
21 cabbage	
1 bundle turnups	25
10 mulberry roots	12

As the Saints became more settled in their new location and adjusted to the conditions of the land upon which they lived, they were able to plant gardens and commence raising their own produce instead of having to live so drastically off the flora and fauna which grew wild in those regions. The unhappy childhood memories of families such as the Hancocks were bettered as these important food supplements became more readily available in the succeeding years. In fact, so successful were their methods of planting, that harvest time yielded generously for some. Mr. Davis records of having made a rather large purchase from one Dr. R.D. Foster[12] sometime in 1842:

20k bushel corn	512 1/2
2 chickens	18
2 bushel potatoes	75

39 bushel corn	85
9 bushel potatoes	337

	$225.00 on acc't
	(Paid him for the same) [13]

It was not until after the Nauvoo expulsion that information becomes more available upon the diet of the Mormon pioneers in regards to "greens." The noted historian Hubert Howe Bancroft mentions of the hardships which they endured that first fall and winter of 1846, in his classic work "The History of Utah":

> *They had not food enough to satisfy the cravings of the sick, nor clothing fit to wear. For months thereafter there were periods when all the flour they used was of the coarser made into hominy. Boiled wheat was now the chief diet for sick and well. For days they subsisted on parched corn. Some mixed their remnant of grain with the pounded BARK of the slippery elm, which they stripped from the trees along their route.*[14]

In fact, the need for raw vegetables and green produce became so acute that several types of dreadful diseases set in among the Mormon people. An eye-witness to these things relates their terrible suffering in these graphic words:

> *In our own journey across the plains, though the time was August, the weather fine, the passage swift, we suffered keenly FROM THE WANT OF FRESH FOOD and of good water. My companion sickened from bile into dysentery... The water almost killed him. His sun-burnt face grew chalky-white; his limbs hung feeble and relaxed; his strong physique so drooped that a man at one of the ranches, after looking at him for a moment with a curious eye, came up to me and said, "you will feel very lonely when he is left behind." My own attack came later, and in another form. The skin of my hands peeled off, as if it had been either frayed or scraped with a knife; boils came out under my back; a pock started on under my eyelid; my fingers had the appearance of scorbutic eruptions.*
>
> *These two diseases, Taylor told me, ravaged the camp of emigrants. Many sickened of dysentery, still more suffered from scurvy.*
>
> *Some of the Saints fell back in the face of these terrible*

> *trials. More fainted by the wayside, and were mournfully laid in their desert graves. Every day there came a funeral, every night there was fresh mourning in the camp. The waste of life is always very great in the emigrant trains... Of the train which I saw come in, six had perished on the plains. But no subsequent train has ever suffered like the first. "The waste of life was great," said Brigham Young, as he told the dreadful tale. Yet the brave, unbroken body of male and female Saints toiled along the frozen way.*[15]

The author of the foregoing narrative mentions, in conclusion, that not until roads were made and the way stations provisioned with FRESH VEGETABLE FOOD, did the toll of death become significantly reduced.

The two most common symptoms of pioneer complaint were dysentery (caused by bad water) and scurvy (caused by a lack of proper greens). For those unfamiliar with the second, an explanation of its conditions is given: "scurvy—Med. A disease characterized by a tendency to hemorrhage, especially into the skin and mucous membranes, and by a spongy condition of the gums, foul breath, loosening of the teeth, anemia, and debility. It results from a lack of vitamin C. *VEGETABLES ARE A SPECIFIC CURE!*"[16]

A constant diet of animal flesh, with little or no produce, will result in some condition of scurvy, in varied extents however, depending upon the individual's consumption pattern in these things. A testimony of this fact is offered by W.C. Staines, an early Mormon missionary who spent a winter among the Ponca Indians while the first small contingency of Saints went westward in search of a new home:

> *Eating, as I had, so much fresh meat WITHOUT VEGETABLES...and having but little exercise, I did not feel as well as I had done, and found a kind of scurvy breaking out on my right side. I had seen something of the kind on some of the Indians, but nothing so bad as mine. All I could do was to apply buffalo fat to the parts affected.*[17]

However, upon remedying his diet with something better, his condition cleared up in almost no time:

> *The third day I felt very faint, and it struck me that if the under bark of the cotton wood tree would feed horses and they could live on it, that it might also serve to stay my hunger. I got*

some young branches, and scraped off a lot of the bark, cutting it fine. I then asked the Lord to bless and sanctify it to my use. I took a mouthful, and after chewing it for some time, swallowed the juice. I was about to swallow the bark, also, when it was suggested to me not to do so, that if I did it would clog my system, but that the juice would not. I therefore, merely chewed the bark, and swallowed only a few mouthfuls of the juice, from which I found relief. For this, and the suggestion not to swallow the bark, I thanked my Heavenly Father.[18]

The evidence is quite plain that when the Saints arrived into the valley of the Great Salt Lake and spent their first several winters here, they had to subsist mainly upon greens. So important was this natural staple to the diet that one of the first injunctions which Brigham Young issued to every newcomer was: "The first duty of a Saint when he comes to this valley, is to learn how to grow *A VEGETABLE*; after which he must learn how to rear pigs and fowls, to irrigate his land, and to build up his house. The rest will come in time."[19] However, the first crops were not too successful. Apostle George A. Smith relates that "a great deal of the grain planted here the first year grew only a few inches high; it was so short it could not be cut. The people had to pull it."[20] Apparently, the same held true for other items also. Some became discouraged and left for the gold mines of California.[21] Bancroft, in his history, mentions that "wild sago and parsnip roots constituted the vegetable food of the settlers. A few deaths occurred from poisonous roots."[22] He further states that because of the "bracing air and hard work" appetites were stimulated which decreased the precious stores of meagre food supply on hand. In the spring, Mr. Bancroft continues, "*THISTLE TOPS* were eaten and became *AN IMPORTANT ARTICLE OF DIET*."[23]

Apostle Parley P. Pratt, in describing those trying times, said: "We toiled hard and lived on a few greens and on thistle and other roots."[24] He further stated, "We had to struggle against great difficulties in trying to mature a first crop." The troubles of which he speaks came about in this interesting manner:

The spring saw everybody busy, and soon there were many flourishing gardens, containing a good variety of vegetables. In the early part of March ploughing commenced. The spring was mild and rain plentiful, and all expected an abundant harvest. But in the latter part of May, when the fields had put on their brightest GREEN, there appeared a visitation in the form of vast swarms of crickets, black and baleful as the locust of the

Dead Sea. In their track they left behind them NOT A BLADE OR LEAF, the appearance of the country which they traversed in countless and desolating myriads being that of a land scorched by fire. They came in a solid phalanx from the direction of Arsenal Hill, darkening the earth in their passage.[25]

Of course, everyone is acquainted with the saving miracle of the seagulls, which preserved a portion and remnant of their precious commodities for that remaining year. "Though the crops of this year of 1848 were thus saved from total destruction, fears were entertained that there would not be food enough for those already in the valley, and the expected arrival of large additional numbers was looked upon as a calamity. The stock of provisions was therefore husbanded with care, many living principally on roots and thistles, to which fare was sometimes added a little flour or milk. The wheat crop, however, turned out better than was expected, and pumpkins, melons, and corn yielded good returns."[26]

Of these times, Apostle Smith said:

"For the next three years we were reduced to considerable straits for food...Rawhides, wolves, rabbits, thistle roots, segoes and everything that could be thought of that would preserve life, were resorted to; there were a few deaths by eating poisonous roots.[27]

Some suffered terribly:

During her pioneer days [Sister R.B. Hill] underwent hardships and suffered many privations,—subsisting on thistle roots, segoes and pigweeds, with a smattering of flour while waging war against grasshoppers and crickets to prevent them from devouring the crops of growing grain and vegetables.[28]

And still others managed along rather nicely:

We [Joseph F. Smith and his mother, Mary Fielding Smith] never lacked so much as many others did; for while we found NETTLE GREENS most acceptable when we first came to the valley, and while WE ENJOYED THISTLE ROOTS, segoes, and all that kind of thing, we were no worse off than thousands of others, and not so bad off as many, for we were never without corn-meal and milk and butter, to my knowledge.[29]

But most of "the people were put upon rations, all sharing the same, like members of one great family. Many, however, in order to swell their scanty store, went out and dug roots with the Indians, or cooked and ate the hides of animals, with which they had covered the roofs of their houses."[30]

This close association with the Lamanite proved invaluable to many early Saints in securing for themselves those "greens" which grew wild in Nature, as the following will prove:

> *While Emily and her relatives were hard put to avoid starvation, it is interesting to note what plants the Indians about her utilized for food, for... they did dry and store mashed seeds of the service berry just as the whites did; but they apparently had a broader knowledge than did the immigrants of the wild flora.*
>
> *They too ate the wild onion (Allium acuminatum), which we find blooming with its rose-purple flowers every May near the present Kaysville cemetery; they too ate the bulbs of the sego lily; but they also used many other plants as well. They ate the cancer root (Orobanche fasciculata), which is parasitic of the sage; and even,* in extreme, *the bitter seeds of the sage itself. They doubtless taught the whites to make bread from the seeds of the sunflower (Relianthus annuus), which grew like a vast yellow field on the present site of Kaysville. They used for chewing gum the spider milkweed or antelope horns (Asolepi-odora decumbena), which we, however, have found growing wild three hundred yards below the mouth of Mill Creek Canyon, some thirty miles south of Emily's home. They also ate the seeds of the more common milkweed (Aeclepias speciosa).*
>
> *Growing along the dry foothills above Kaysville is the "big sunflower" big root or arrow-leaved balsam root (Baiearn-orrhiza sagittata) with broad yellow flowers. The Indians ate its leaves as greens, and later its seeds. It is a low perennial herb, not at all like the common sunflower (Helianthus annuua). They also used rabbit brush (Chrysothamnus graveolens) for chewing gum.*
>
> *Several species of the genus Opuntia, prickly pears or cacti, grew in the valley that to Emily was home; and the Indians thereabout were smart enough to burn off the spines and eat the partially cooked body, sometimes roots as well. They treated the thistle (Cirsium undulatum) in the same manner...*

On moist mountain slopes next to receding snow in March we have found blooming a delightful pink flower four inches high, known as spring beauty (Claytonia rosea), the Indians ate its roots, especially of the species Claytonia megarrhiaa.

Wild rye (Elymus condensatus), which grows from three to six feet high, along the dry foothills and mountainsides above Kaysville, bears grains, which the Indians gathered and made into flour.

Often when we traverse the gravelly hillsides above Kaysville in early March we come upon a yellow flowered perennial, which is like a small mat on the ground, blooming before anything else seems ready, it is the Indian parsnip (Aulospermum longipes), a member of the carrot or parsley family, the thick roots of which the Indians ate. Almost at the same time appears that delightful little flower, the buttercup (Fritillaria pudica), whose blooms are like thimbles of rich yellow butter. Many is the time we have joyfully gathered them, but the less aesthetic Indians pulled and ate their bulbs; for like the onions and sego lilies they are members of the lily family. While we are on this subject we should mention that alongside the wild onions, the sego lilies and the dogtooth violets, there grows another member of the Liliaceas known as the star lily, death camas or poison sego (Zigadenus elegane), the bulbs of which are so poisonous that they have caused many deaths among uninformed people innocently mistaking them for the delicious "sego lily," the state flower of Utah...

They ate the seeds of a goosefoot (Chenopodium rubrum) that grew over a foot high in alkaline or even salty soil near Emily's home, and made tea from mint, as did the whites. The Indians got their sugar from the common reed (Phragmitea communis), the stalks and roots of which they gathered and ground into a flour, which when heated tasted like the marshmallow of the present day.

Watercress (Radicula pacifica and allied species) was gathered everywhere by Indians for salad; but for some reason it was not cultivated much in England a century ago, and the pioneers made but casual use of it. I have never tried it dried; but certainly it grows in every spring and cold brook in the Kaysville region...

Indians used for food not only the sego lily and wild onion but also another member of the lily family known as the camas (Camassia quamash), a perennial with globose bulbs, which grows in wet meadows. It was a much more common food in Idaho than near the Great Salt Lake, where it was usually gathered, baked and made into large cakes that were sweet like molasses. It grows in wet meadows near Kaysville, but apparently it was used more by the Weber Utes in their northern homes..

The upshot of the matter is, that one need not starve if he knows his flora and is as wise as the chipmunk, which at least puts edible bits aside to dry for future use.[31]

One sometimes is led to wonder just how the pioneers would have fared without their red man brother to assist them, as they dug for their survival in Nature's produce.

Eating this type of humble fare seemed disgraceful to some, and delightful to others.

At times provisions were scarce in the valley. Brother John went digging pepper mint roots, which greatly humbled him, together with patched britches. When he left Zion he never returned. Preferred to stay in the land of plenty. Milk weed shoots, early in the spring were considered luscious. Any kind of greens were sought after. One day, I picked young early marrowfat peas, and young green currants and started for Bishop Callister. Got Helen Mar, his wife, interested. She dug early beets, radishes, and some other garden vegetables.

One day there was nothing to eat at the farm. Mother Williams rode up the surry, to see if I had received from those who had promised to pay me the Bill they were owing Dr. Williams. None had paid. I had just arrived at the house as she drove up with an osnebery [?] sack holding a bushel and a half of young beet greens, Brother Kimball Tucker helping me. When Mother Williams saw them her eyes sparkled. She was particularly fond of anything to eat with vinegar. She wanted half; I gave her all, as they had to work in the hot sun and wanted something to keep up their strength to work on. Sister Vilate sent 4 pounds of pork to cook which was a treat to the ploughmen and sowers of grain and corn. I continued to pick weeds with the milk they brought from the farm and skim milk Mrs. Hyde gave me. I lived around all that to be 71 years old, though I was 28 at that time of life, not knowing of the future.[31a]

Today's modern housewife in Utah generally goes to the local supermarket to do her shopping for the green things which her family needs for their health and sustenance. However, the early female Saint secured hers another way:

> *The time had come when the work was to be done, and I had not one day's rations to commence with. However, the nettles were up about three inches, so for food I resorted to them. I would get up very early and go and hunt the oxen, then go to the nettle bed, and gather my breakfast, stew the greens in salty water and then eat them. When dinner time came I went through the same operation. Sometimes I obtained a little butter from some good sister to grease my greens with.*[32]

However, it appears that the Saints still remaining in Winter Quarters, and other locales, fared better with a more balanced diet of domestic produce than what their Utah comrades did. An examination of a tithing account, paid in kind by one Edwin Harley, who resided on Mosquito Creek, in 1848, reveals a variety of items with which he gave his "ten percent to the Lord":

Amount of produce raised in 1848

60	bushels	potatoes
210	bushels	corn
44	bushels	buckwheat
6	bushels	turnips
2	bushels	beets
30	chickens	
10	dozen eggs	

1848 Tything payed to Bishop G. Snow

6	bushels	potatoes
21	bushels	corn
4	bushels	buckwheat
1/2	bushels	turnips
1/4	bushels	beets
3	chickens	
1	dozen eggs.	

Apparently, the good brother felt that the Lord was not partial to turnips and beets and therefore held back a little more than what he should have done, lest these two greens find no favor with the Almighty. But the record basically shows what they grew at these Mormon encampments, which certainly seems an improvement upon what they were trying to raise (?) out West.

Parley P. Pratt made the observation, though, that despite their hardships experienced that first winter, the year of 1848 was deemed a "pretty good year," after all things were taken into consideration:

> *On the 10th of August we held a public feast under a bowery in the centre of our fort. This was called a harvest feast; we partook freely of a rich variety of bread, beef, butter, cheese, cakes, pastry, green corn, melons, and ALMOST EVERY VARIETY OF VEGETABLE. Large sheaves of wheat, rye, barley, oats and other productions were hoisted on poles for public exhibition, and there was prayer and thanksgiving, congratulations, songs, speeches, music, dancing, smiling faces and merry hearts. In short, it was a great day with the people of these valleys, and long to be remembered by those who had suffered and waited anxiously for the results of a first effort to redeem the interior deserts of America, and to make her hitherto unknown solitudes "blossom as the rose."*[34]

And again, in '49, they had an occasion to rival the one of the year previous:

> *The 24th of July was a day long to be remembered by all present in this valley, and all Saints who shall learn of our celebration, as the anniversary of the arrival of the Pioneers two years previous. To behold twelve or fifteen hundred feet of tables, filling the bowery and all adjoining grounds, loaded with all luxuries of the field and gardens, and NEARLY ALL THE VARIETIES THAT ANY VEGETABLE MARKET IN THE WORLD COULD PRODUCE, and to see the seats around those tables filled and re-filled by a people who had been deprived of those luxuries for years by the cruel hand of oppression...was a theme of unbounded thanks giving and praise to the Giver of all good...*[35]

So it seems that despite the inclement odds against them, they somehow managed in the face of it all. And what is still more interesting is the fact that from such a diet of greens and wholesome, nutritous vegetables, their health generally increased and became better, and there was no disease to be found among them whatsoever. The First Presidency of the Church at that time (Brigham Young, Heber C. Kimball, and Willard Richards) verified this with a public statement issued abroad to all the Saints in the world: "The health of the Saints in the valley is good, and it is so seldom that anyone dies, we scarce recollect when such an event last occurred."[36] No wonder Brigham Young was led to remark some years later, when the people had grown rather corpulent and contented from the fat of the land: "I sometimes think we were better off what we did, when we first came here."[37]

About that same time, he gave the Saints an injunction to follow, which stressed the need in the Mormon diet of what we have been talking about: "...vegetables are good and healthful. But vegetables are not grown among us as they should be; there is not that attention paid to them that, it seems to me, they should receive. My theory is, that if we wish to raise a healthy, noble-looking, intellectual and perfect race of men and women, *WE MUST FEED OUR CHILDREN PROPERLY.*"[38] And green vegetables was *HIGH ON THE LIST* of what the Prophet had in mind.

President George A. Smith, counselor to Brigham Young, was also quick to point up the importance of such things in one's daily menu:

> *If men wish to grow up in these mountains, FREE FROM DISEASE, and from the power of the destroyer, and become STRONG AND POWERFUL LIKE TIGERS—like GIANTS IN ISRAEL, let them observe the principles laid down in the words of wisdom, let them observe them when they are children, let them grow up breathing a pure atmosphere, drinking pure water, and PARTAKING OF THE WHOLESOME VEGE TATION, observing the words of wisdom, and they will grow up mighty men.*[39]

And a noted American medical specialist in the twentieth century, Dr. Victor Heiser, recognized internationally for his efforts to benefit mankind, had similar views upon the same subject in our time:

> *The cauliflower is the vegetable which contains calcium in greatest quantities...*
>
> *When I was young my parents had no knowledge of vitamins and mineral salts. They both had bad teeth; so did I. By the time I was sixteen I complained of suffering from toothache and received the sage advice, "Why not go to a dentist?" But that art had not been developed very far. I still recall the little show-*

case filled with false teeth that was displayed with dentist street signs. With better dentistry and knowledge of nutrition, much could have been done for me. In those days I ate NO LEAFY VEGETABLES at all. I did not like them. And my teeth began to go to pieces. But when I changed my food habits the decay stopped, although I admit this may have had something to do with my age.

It is highly desirable to INCLUDE RAW VEGETABLES IN THE DIET. They digest fairly easily unless they contain too much cellulose; only the hardy can contend with the turnip. Carrots are good and the necessary chewing actions helps preserve the teeth. If you are unable for dental reasons to cope with raw carrots in the large, grating them is a simple matter and removes the frequent objection to the tough fibers.

A salad composed of celery, cauliflower, spinach, lettuce, potatoes, green peas, almonds, tomatoes, and a seasoning of salt would contain all the necessary mineral salts in abundance. Although many salad vegetables are too expensive for some families in winter, yet they are essential, and among Chinese cabbage, chives, endive, escarole, lettuce, romaine, watercress, some should be found to meet the purse...

Wherever you are, whatever your income, YOU SHOULD HAVE LEAFY VEGETABLES IN YOUR DIET![40]

In the light of such sound advice from men of God and honorable men of the earth, how can Latter-day Saints continue to ignore the laws of decent health, and the promising youth of Zion so casually wink at good nutrition by their careless and abusive eating habits? Should they continue in their downward trend, the Apostle Paul's prophetic words shall invariably be fulfilled upon their foolish heads: "*WHATSOEVER A MAN SOWETH, THAT SHALL HE ALSO REAP.*"[41]

It is a curious thing in our history that when the early Saints were in want of food God provided them with greens as a general rule, instead of the common commodities of flesh and fowl, though there are on record a few instances of the latter, too. But it is with the former that He seems to have been more generous in providing them, as the following two accounts go to prove:

In 1855, the grasshoppers made their appearance in the settlements in Utah and did much damage. They took all of the crops and garden stuff of Grandfather Hemingway, except a small patch of garden peas about twenty feet square. The family gathered roots and pig greens and anything else to help out the food supply. Each morning grandmother would go to this patch of peas and carefully pick every pea, about enough for a scant meal. She would say, "I have picked every pea—these are the last, what will we do now?"—and grandfather would reply—"The Lord will provide for us." Each morning she would go to the pea patch and get just enough for another meal and say "Now this is the last"—but on the morn there would be just enough for another meal. This continued for weeks and really kept them alive.[42]

* * *

The following story is told by Abigail Cox Heaton, whose parents were among the first sent to colonize Manti, Utah:

When her father and mother moved first to Manti, they built their dugout at the foot of the hill on which the Manti Temple now stands. At first they had a fair supply of food, but later, like the rest of the territory, the droughts left them almost in the throes of famine. For one summer, they had little else than greens, and finally even the supply of greens was exhausted. There were many families in the Valley, and the women and children scoured the land for greens.

One day, Mrs. Heaton's brother, Walter Cox, had hunted most of the afternoon with little luck. The few spindly weeds were scarcely enough for one person, let alone for a family of five or seven, and the children were crying for food. Walter himself was only a young boy. People prayed in humility for something to eat.

Next morning, Mother Cox gave Walter the basket and told him to go in search of greens. It was useless, he told her, for they could find none the day before. But she reminded him of their prayers, and that the Lord had never utterly deserted them. She knelt with her children in prayer then started Walter off. Almost hopeless, but willing to do his part and obey his mother, Walter began his search.

In an amazingly short time he returned to the dugout with a basket of such crisp, stalky greens, even his mother was amazed. He was almost breathless as he told her of having found a large patch of the luscious weeds, just as if they had been planted in rows, and on the same ground where many had been searching the day previous. Never had they eaten such good greens, and for days the people of the Manti Valley gathered baskets of greens that seemed to satisfy their hunger and even some claimed, put flesh on them. Almost before their eyes, another miracle had happened, for it was as if the green had come up over night.

Mrs. Heaton is now along in years, but often recalls how their mother used to remind them of this incident, whenever they seemed to question life or lack faith.[43]

In such precarious times, when reliance seemed to be placed more upon God than upon man, the Latter-day Saints enjoyed an outpouring of the gifts of the Spirit. Such unique features as tongues, the interpretation of tongues, open visions and realistic prophecies were not uncommon with the people then. And, like our first parents in the garden, they enjoyed a spiritual bliss which twentieth century rationalization does not seem to offer these days. For we read in the Good Book that Adam "walked and talked with God" while living in Eden. Now, the question arises, "Why was he able to do this so easily?" The simple answer would seem to be "he had not yet sinned." But a more careful examination of scripture will always reveal that *HIS DIET* had a lot to do with it, too.

Now, to some this may seem silly, but the purported absurdity which some may entertain in regards to this thought is quickly dismissed from some statements of President Brigham Young. Upon one occasion, in Cedar City, "Brigham said he believed the Saints eat too much too enjoy the spirit."[44] And at still another time he remarked, "Let me have something that will sustain Nature and leave my stomach and whole system clear to *RECEIVE THE SPIRIT OF THE LORD*, and be free from head ache and pains of every kind.... The vegetable kingdom is made for man, to gratify the taste and *ADD HEALTH TO THE BODY* and gratification to every sense."[45]

Greens and vegetables are easy to digest. Medical science will tell you that. While their opposites of heavy meat and sweet pastries tend to clog the system and jam the digestive tract. And the body has to work twice or three times as hard to properly assimilate these things. Greens are so much easier and more pleasant for the body to handle.

Thus, we can see from the previous assertion that Adam's diet in the Garden, which consisted mainly of nuts, and berries, and the herbs of the field, had a lot to do with what he was able to enjoy in the realm of spiritual blessings. Not until after his expulsion from Eden did he develop a subsequent habit for flesh. And then we find that his contacts with the Lord became less frequent and more effort was required on his part to keep in touch with the Almighty than what had been heretofore.

Now, wc arc not advocating strict vegetarianism when this point is discussed. For the Lord said a great truth that "whoso forbiddeth to abstain from meats, that man should not eat the same, *IS NOT ORDAINED OF GOD.*"[46] Such a pernicious doctrine is of the Devil, and there are those among us who would have some of the weaker believe that an all-vegetable diet is the proper thing in order to achieve great spiritual success. But, this is not in accord with the revealed will of God, nor in harmony with what His servants, such as Brigham Young, have said upon the subject.

President Young merely stressed that overeating reduces our awareness. And that by maintaining a sensible diet, which would include simple greens of nourishing value, our stomachs and entire systems would be left free and clear to enjoy the wonderful Spirit of God in richer abundance. Certainly they that love the Lord should adopt this as a practice to follow, in order to achieve greater things for themselves and their families in days to come.

And finally, the importance of greens may be given in terms of "future survival" for those of us who will go to the trouble and time to learn about these things and hunt them up in the times of our greatest need.

> *"I see men, women and children standing and sometimes sitting in the streets, bare footed and bare-headed and crying for food; and they will often follow me eight or ten rods begging for food. Ninety thousand people have come from Ireland to the city of Liverpool alone, to get food and employment. The multitudes that die from starvation are so numerous in places in Ireland that they are not even buried at all, but straw and grass are thrown over them and they rot above ground. More factories are stopping every day, and more and more people are thrown out of employment, and emigration is so great that there are not ships enough to take the emigrants. Freight and passage are very high and rising. Universal fear and consternation pervade England, Ireland, and France, and many other parts of Europe."*[47]

No! Such a thing was not a fearful vision of an Orwellian future, as seen by some early member of the Church. Rather instead, it was a very real account of a dramatic situation experienced by Elder Orson Spencer in Liverpool, England in April of 1847. Yet the horrible realities of his past could very well become our present future in no time at all.

Included with this work, in the appendix section, Part II, is a list of nutritive plants and their value, plus short recommendations as to their use. The reader is kindly referred to them, at his convenience, to study and peruse in leisure.

In conclusion, it may be asked, "What is the purpose for cultivating such a taste for the edible plants of the earth?" And, it can very well be answered in this manner: at the commencement of the Millennium all flesh which is dependent upon meat for part of its diet shall have lost that craving for such carnal things. This includes both man and beast alike. Proof of this is offered by the great Prophet Isaiah:

> *The wolf shall dwell with the lamb, and the leopard shall lie down with the kid; and the calf and the young lion and the fatling together; and a little child shall lead them.*
>
> *And the cow and the bear shall feed; their young ones shall lie down together, and the LION SHALL EAT STRAW LIKE THE OX!*
>
> *They SHALL NOT HURT NOR DESTROY in all my holy mountain...*
>
> *And again:*
>
> *The wolf and the lamb shall FEED TOGETHER, and the LION SHALL EAT STRAW LIKE THE BULLOCK; and dust shall be the serpent's meat. They SHALL NOT HURT NOR DESTROY in all my holy mountain, saith the Lord.*[48]

What further evidence does one need than this? He clearly tells us how it shall be with both. Or, in other words, conditions shall be then, as they were in Adam's day, and man shall eat of the good things in the garden, that he might walk and talk with his Maker as our first progenitor did so long ago.

Yet despite such accurate predictions there will always be those who remain somewhat dubious over the matter in discussion. For them, scripture is not good enough; for they believe a man has read his own interpretation into the thing. They must have bona fide authority in order to accept it as doctrine. So, to satisfy their disgruntled views, a "living oracle" is quoted. Elder Orson Pratt, an Apostle of the Lord Jesus Christ in the latter days, expressed the transition from carnal appetite to natural taste, in these appropriate words:

> *This change will be wrought upon ALL FLESH when Jesus comes; not a change to immortality, but a change sufficient to alter the ferocious Nature of beast, birds and fishes. In those days the lion will eat straw like the ox; he will no more be the terror of the forest, but will be perfectly harmless, and gentleness will characterize all the wild and ferocious animals, as well as the venomous serpents, so much so that the little child might lead them and play with them, and nothing should hurt or destroy in all the holy mountain of the Lord; all things becoming, in some measure, as when they were first created. For it will be remembered that animals did not devour one another until after the fall, neither was there any death, until after the fall. What did they eat, then? The Lord said, "To every beast of the field, and to every thing that creepeth upon the earth, wherein there is life, I have given every green herb for meat." The grass, and the herbs, and every green thing were their food. And ADAM AND EVE ATE FRUITS AND VEGETABLES, NOT ANIMAL FLESH. The whole earth will be restored; and MAN WILL BE RESTORED; and not only upon man, but upon all flesh the Spirit of God will be poured out and THEY WILL eventually BE RESTORED TO ALL THAT WAS LOST BY THE FALL OF OUR FIRST PARENTS!*[49]

And, if the law of tithing should still be in existence then, conditions of payment similar to Brigham Young's time shall prevail in that day, also:

> *We went next to the Tithing House, inside the buttressed wall of which I have spoken. Here, within separate courts devoted to different articles, the faithful are supposed to devote one tenth of what they raise or receive to the support of the Church. Loads of hay were driven into one yard. Some new spring-carriages stood under a shed. There was a long row of vegetable cellars opening by hatches under a sort of porch; in this were rooms with counters which looked like the obscure shops in the suburbs of great cities, such as one might find at Harlem or South Boston. Counters were set a little way within the doors. At each was a man with an account book, who wrote down what*

was deceived.[50]

What finer thing could a man offer than, when it is asked of him, "What do you have to offer the Lord this day?" and he can proudly say, "*SOME GREENS I GREW MYSELF.*"

NOTES

1. Genesis 3:24.

2. *Webster's New International Dictionary*, 2nd Ed. Unabridged, Mass., 1946; p. 2823.

3. Leah D. Widstoe, *How To Be Well*; Missouri, 1943; p. 284.

4. *JD* 20:18

5. Diary of Charles L. Walker, p. 741; Special Collections, Harold B. Lee Library, Brigham Young University, Provo, Utah.

6. Genesis 25:27—29; 34.

7. Genesis 34:24—29.

8. Genesis 47:28.

9. D & C 89:10.

10. *JD* 12:118—119.

11. *The Mosiah Hancock Journal*—Life Story; privately published; no place or date of publication given, nor company mentioned; available at Zion's Book Store, Salt Lake; pp. 13—14.

12. A scribe of Joseph Smith's, and personal acquaintance, who later turned against the Prophet, apostatized, and became one of his bitterest foes thereafter.

13. Amos David, *op., cit.* (previous chapter notes).

14. Hubert Howe Bancroft, *History of Utah*; p. 233.

15. William Hepworth Dixon, *New America;* Philadelphia, 1867: pp. 164—165.

16. Webster's, *op., cit.*, p. 2252.

17. *A String Of Pearls—Second Book of The Faith-Promoting Series*; Salt Lake, 1880; p. 17.

18. *Ibid.*, p. 20.

19. Dixon, *op., cit.*, p. 166.

20. *JD* 13:120.

21. *Ibid.*

22. Bancroft, *op., cit.*, p. 176.

23. *Ibid.*

24. *The Autobiography of Parley Parker Pratt*, by Parley Parker Pratt; New York, 1874; pp. 405-6.

25. Bancroft, *op., cit.*, pp. 279-280.

26. *Ibid.*, p. 282.

27. *JD* 13:120.

28. Dr. Daniel B. Hill Richards, *Hill Family History*; Salt Lake, 1927; p. 55.

29. Joseph Fielding Smith, *Life of Joseph F. Smith*; Salt Lake, 1938; p. 159.

30. *Preston Nibley, Faith Promoting Stories*; Missouri, 1943; p. 28.

31. Claude T. Barnes, *The Grim Years Or The Life of Emily Stewart Barnes*; Kaysville, Utah, 1964; pp. 38—41.

3la. Account Book of Frederick G. Williams, pp. 237-238—239-240. Church Historian Office, Salt Lake City.

32. Nibley, *op., cit.*, p. 89.

33. Journal of Edwin Harly, Book One, 1848. Harold B. Lee Library, BYU, Provo.

34. Pratt, *op., cit.*, p. 406.

35. *The Frontier Guardian* (Kanesville, Iowa), December 26, 1849.

36. *Ibid.*

37. Material in author's possession.

38. *JD* 12:223.

39. *JD* 2:363.

40. Victor Heiser, M.D., *You're The Doctor*; New York, 1939; pp. 96–98.

41. Galatians 6:7.

42. Written by their granddaughter, Elvira D. Ballard; as appeared in the DUP Lesson for May, 1941, p. 343, by Kate B. Carter.

43. *Ibid*, pp. 344–345.

44. Journal of Jacob Hamblin, p. 20.

45. *JD* 13:153; 8:82.

46. D & C 49:18.

47. Barnes, *op., cit.*, p. 8.

48. Isaiah 11:6–9; 65:25.

49. *JD* 20:18.

50. Caroline H. Dall, *My First Holiday*; Boston, 1881; p. 94.

CHAPTER THREE

MILK IS A NATURAL

(Joseph Smith and Dairy Products)

Surprising as it may seem to some, the common liquid of milk was a favorite with at least four Presidents of the Church. Together with stone-ground whole wheat bread, Prophets Joseph Smith, Brigham Young, Wilford Woodruff, and Joseph Fielding Smith relished this humble fare more than they did any other substance available.

Beginning with Brother Joseph, we find him occasionally complaining when Emma would set MORE than just these two items before him.

> *"When I want a little bread and milk," he said once to William W. Phelps, when the two were dining alone at the Prophet's home, "my wife loads the table with so many good things, IT DESTROYS MY APPETITE!"*[1]

Joseph Smith did not care for big meals as such. Oh, on certain occasions and special celebrations, such as Christmas, he would allow his wife to go 'all out,' and prepare a table of those same 'good things,' which she was so fond of creating to please him. As with all good women who love to cook, Emma thought that "the way to a man's heart was through his stomach." Hence, the numerous dinners of full-course meals. But what she did not realize was that he understood the laws of health better than she did, and being a plain and simple man by Nature, took delight in plain and simple things, such as home-made bread and good raw milk.

At another time, when he had a group of men working for him splitting rails and invited them in to eat with his family, we find that that particular meal consisted of only those things which he loved the most:

> *"When noon came we were all called to dinner at Joseph's house. The table was loaded down with corn-meal mush AND MILK, and at the bidding of Joseph we all stepped forward to our places around the table, standing on our feet. Joseph*

asked Joshua F. Holman, who was one of the wood haulers, to ask the blessing on the food. He went at his duty with all his soul. As he had been a Methodist exhorter before joing the Church, he commenced to call upon the great and mighty God who sat upon the top of a topless throne, to look down and bless the food and asked many other blessings to rest upon the Prophet, etc.

As soon as he closed, Brother Joseph said, "Brother Joshua, don't let me ever hear you ask another such a blessing." And then before we took our seats he stated his reasons for making this remark, and showed us how inconsistent such ideas were, and told us many things about God and who He was. Then we sat down to our mush AND MILK..."[2]

In fact, so used to milk was he, that the Prophet would often allude to it in parables used to illustrate some principle of the Gospel better:

I recollect very distinctly hearing the Prophet Joseph say that the kingdom had come, but the will was not done yet on the earth as it was done in heaven; and in order that the sisters especially might understand it, he said, "You sisters can understand it by this little similitude. When you scald out your milk pans, you have the milk pan." "Yes." "But it is not full of milk?" "No, of course not." "Now, here the kingdom has come, but His will is not done on earth, yet as it is done in heaven. The milkpan is not filled up yet in doing the will of God." We are here to learn and to toil to this end; not only those who are grey-haired and bald-headed, but the boys and girls. It is for all of us to do the works of righteousness and faith, that the will of God may be done on earth as it is done in heaven, so that there may not only be a milkpan, but a pan of milk. I heard the Prophet make use of this figure in the grove at the top of the hill, just in front of where the temple stood, in Nauvoo.[3]

As to the value and usefulness of milk in the human system, the noted American physician of the late 1930's, Dr. Victor Heiser, had this to say about it:

Milk is practically a perfect food, lacking only sufficient iron. It includes in proper proportions the five requisites—proteins, fats, carbohydrates, vitamins, and minerals. In fact, with the exception of leafy vegetables, it alone will supply the deficiencies in cereals, tubers, and other foodstuffs, which so often lead to disorder or disease.[4]

Between the constant advertising on television and many medical men's views, milk is believed to be the best thing for all-around nourishment. To some degree, this may hold true. But to interpret the above opinion of Dr. Heiser to mean that this dairy product itself will suffice, is wrong and not consistent with the basic teachings of Joseph Smith upon the matter.

Hyrum Smith, brother to the Prophet, had a little boy, Joseph by name. As he grew up he was weaned on nothing but this substance, with very little of anything else included in his diet. The following circumstance was the result of several years feeding him this way, and brought about the suggestion from the Prophet in regards to better nutrition for the boy all around:

> *I saw him and my father as they were rowed in a skiff across the Mississippi river, and watched them till they landed at the bank of the river near the old Times and Seasons printing office, and watched them as they walked up the bank of the river on to Water Street, and walked along and came into our house. Joseph sat down while my father washed and arranged his toilet. And while Uncle Joseph was sitting there, he took me on his knee and tottered me and played with me. In a little while my father came in. Joseph says, "What is the matter with this little boy?" Father said, "Nothing, I guess." He says, "He looks as though he hadn't a drop of blood in him." I remember it so well. Up to this time, you may remember, I had lived on milk, a good deal of it skim milk, and I suppose I was rather pale—a circumstance that arose through the prostrated condition of my mother, brought on by cruel persecutions in Missouri.*[5]

The Prophet "then advised that he be fed a little more solid food."[6]

Drinking skim milk as consistently as what the boy had done, is not good enough to provide one with all of the proper nourishment his body needs. Other things, such as more solids, are necessary in order to bring a balance and harmony in one's diet. Though the processes of pasteurization and homogenization were unknown in those days, yet "skimming" was a common thing, in order to preserve the rich cream for other uses. Good, fresh, whole raw milk was what the Saints drank in those days, and the benefits derived from this enormous consumption seemed to be more lasting than present day milk. People then drank a wholesome substance of something good. Our modern-day technology has conveniently removed the best part for hygenic reasons, and given us a liquified pablum as the final result. So what the state Board of Health may say is safe for consumption is not necessarily nourishing for good nutrition.

But even in the good old days, problems could arise from skimming:

> *While in Far West, I was at the trial of Sister Marsh, the wife of Thomas B. Marsh. He was President of the Twelve; for skimming milk. Several sisters in Far West had agreed to unite in making cheese by putting their milk together. Each one promised not to skim their milk. The trial was before Bishop Edward Partridge, where it was proved that she had not kept her promise and was about to withdraw the hand of fellowship. The Bishop and others plead with her to make things right and offered her time to do so. But no, for she called on God and angels to witness her innocence. At this, the Prophet jumped up and said, "Sister Marsh, if you say that you lie like the Devil!" This remark from the Prophet at that time made me stare. However, on a little reflection, I soon got over it.*[7]

Though it is very doubtful that any big concerns these days will ever be brought to trial for "skimming the best off the top" as Sister Marsh did, yet it would be interesting to know just what Joseph Smith would say to them, if they protested that their homogenized and pastuerized product was as good as what came straight from the cow. Being a man of truth, he certainly did not mince words with the lady. Would the claims of the dairy corporations fare any better under his honest scrutiny?

In the Millennial Star, Elder William D. McAllister made this remark about milk:

> *Milk is one of the most necessary foods in the human diet as is proved in every country by countless experiments. Its use is imperative for children. But it is a food and not a drink; and should be eaten slowly. It is one of our best sources of protein, and is the chief so-called "protective food."*[8]

As a reliable food source, then, many of the early Latter-day Saints depended upon this substance for their mainstay of nourishment at times. This was usually in times of recovery from illness, or in dire hardship. Elijah Fordham had been near death's door at Commerce, Illinois, in 1839, when the Prophet, in company with others, visited him:

> *Joseph stood erect, still holding his hand in silence several moments; then he spoke in a very loud voice, saying, "Brother Fordham, I command you, in the name of Jesus Christ, to arise from this bed and be made whole." His voice was like the voice of God, and not of man. It seemed as though the house shook to its very foundations. Brother Fordham arose from his bed and was immediately made whole. His feet were bound in poultices which he kicked off; then putting on his clothes, he ate A BOWL OF BREAD AND MILK and followed the Prophet into the street.*[9]

Even those who had been on the other side visiting friends and loved ones found a common dish such as this to their particular liking, once they returned to good old "terra firma":

> *As soon as the brethren had taken their hands from his head he raised up in bed, sitting erect, and in another moment turned his legs off the bed.*
>
> *At this juncture Joseph asked him if he had not better be careful, for he was very weak. He replied, 'I never felt better in my life,' almost immediately adding, 'I want my pants.'*
>
> *His pants were found and given him, which he drew on, Joseph assisting him, although he thought he needed no help. Then he signified his intention to sit in a chair at or near the fire-place. Joseph took hold of his arm to help him along safely, but William declared his ability to walk alone, notwithstanding which, the help continued.*
>
> *Astonishment had taken the place of weeping throughout the room. Every looker-on was ready to weep for joy; but none were able or felt inclined to talk, Presently William said he wanted some thing to eat. Joseph asked him what he would like, and he replied that he wanted A DISH OF BREAD AND MILK.*
>
> *Emma immediately brought what he called for, as one may easily comprehend, every hand was anxious to supply the wants of a man who, a few moments before was dead, really and truly dead! Brother Huntington ate the BOWL OF BREAD AND MILK with as good a relish as any he ever ate.*[10]

And President Wilford Woodruff found more nourishment and strength in "ole bossy's" yield than he did in anything else when sick:

> *May 6 (1893) Saturday. The President passed a good night. He ate a small bowl of bread and MILK AND DRANK THREE TUMBLERS OF MILK (besides)! He seems quite right; has no pain. I am quite hopeful for him. If he will only exert his faith, he can get well and live...*[11]

During the historic trek across the plains in 1848 by the mass of thousands of emigrants, food was a serious problem:

> *That five thousand persons, including a very large proportion of women and children, almost without money, almost without provisions, except THE MILK of their kine and the grain which they had raised near their own camps, should, almost without the loss of a life, have accomplished this journey of more than twelve hundred miles, crossing range after range of mountains, bridging rivers, and traversing deserts, while liable at any moment to be attached by roaming bands of savages, is one of the marvels that this century has witnessed!*[12]

The late President Joseph Fielding Smith loved this as his favorite dairy product also. According to his late wife, Jessie Evans, "Homemade bread is a favorite food of President Smith. On Thursday evenings he traditionally has a supper of bread and milk with slices of nippy cheese."[13]

Cheese was another staple of early Mormon diet, and could be found in their households quite frequently. Captain James Brown, in writing home of his family, reminds them in a letter of February 22, 1854: "Do the best you all can. Raise good gardens; plenty pigs and chickens. Make some GOOD CHEESE and have it mellowing...."[14] Another pioneer recalls this experience in her girlhood: "Making cheese was always the most interesting to me, seeing the curd set and how the presser pressed it down so solidly and how the big wheel just turned around to press the weight down."[15]

Apparently this must have been a favorite food with the Lord, for, when two of His servants, on an occasion once asked him for something to eat, He had His angels provide them with this, in the following remarkable manner:

It was in the Spring of the year 1844, when many of the best men in the Church were out on a special mission, to advocate the election of the Prophet Joseph Smith to the Presidency of the United States, that my father, Bishop Hoagland, was traveling with Elder George A. Smith, stomping the country for this purpose. They were traveling in a light one-horse wagon, taking their chances with the people, for their food and lodgings. One day, when they had gone without necessary accommodations too long, they both felt much in need of something to eat. They had entered a small patch of timber, where there was some nice, green grass, when Elder George A. Smith, said: "Let us stop here and ask the Lord for something to eat—here is plenty for the horse." This suggestion was at once carried out. The horse was unhitched and let out on the grass, while the brethren retired into a more secluded place and engaged in prayer, especially asking for something to satisfy their hunger. After prayer they felt entirely satisfied as far as the cravings of their stomachs were concerned, and after a while they hitched up and proceeded on their journey, but they had only gone a very short distance, when they were surprised by finding A LARGE CHEESE lying upon a stone in the middle of the road and a clean new knife lying crossways on the top of it. Brother Smith said, "Here is our supper," and so they stopped and, with thankful hearts, proceeded on their journey, taking the cheese with them.[16]

Brigham Young's favorite dish was "a little clabbered milk and some johnny-cake." Often he would wish for this, when everything else of a delectable Nature would be laid before him. Now some of the more petite may turn their noses up at such a sour concoction, but medically-speaking, it is one of the best things for a person:

The souring of milk is a perfectly natural process caused by the lactic acid bacilli which feed on the milk sugar. Sour milk, good and thick, flavored with cinnamon and sweetened with sugar, makes a delectable food. It tends to compensate for the failure of the stomach to secrete enough hydrochloric acid, and is excellent therefore for those over forty. The process of souring also kills off many undesirable bacteria and predigests certain caseins that those with weak digestions might not be able to handle.[17]

The author remembers an experience he had with sour milk last summer quite by accident. He had left his Manti residence and gone to Salt Lake upon some very important business. He took along two gallons of fresh goat's milk with him. He stayed for several days at his aunt and uncle's place, while he conducted his business in that city. The first gallon of milk he consumed in one day. The second, however, he let sit a few days longer in an extra refrigerator in the basement. It kept the liquid cool, yet not enough, for the stuff began to turn and commence clabbering. The month was July, and the weather extremely hot!

Coming home that particular evening, he discovered the change in the contents, but decided rather than to discard it, to let the aging process continue. Several days afterwards, when the substance was thick and juicy like cottage cheese, he removed it from the bottle and had himself several helpings of it.

The smell was unbearable, but sufficient honey over the top made it quite a pleasant and tasty item to chew contently on.

But the ironic part was that shortly after his pleasurable repast, his aunt came downstairs to get something from the fruit room. The table had been cleared and all appearances of a previous meal there had been eliminated. He will never forget how she sniffed the air different times, and the quizzical expression which appeared upon her face as she asked the author, "John—what is that smell in the basement?" He did not have the heart nor the courage to tell her what it was, so assumed it could be a gas leak in the line somewhere, perhaps. However, she knew better, though unable to identify precisely what it was.

Several days later, he informed her of the correct Nature of that peculiar odor, and she pulled a long grimace of expression in reply to it. But for himself, the author must say that he found the resulting concoction quite pleasant and enjoyable, when sweetened with something. Some, however, would gag on this sort of thing, if not used to it. Now, the author is not in the habit of eating such a dish as this, and leaves it for another time, when the food economy may not be able to provide him with that which his palate is adjusted to. But, the experience of that hot summer day will long be remembered as one of the healthiest nourishments he has ever partaken of.

Similar episodes in pioneer times had a way of making people wonder, too—even to such an extent as almost breaking up a marriage before the day's wedding had ended:

> *Nearly three years passed, and having made all preparations for his life partner, Loce took the trail back to Farmington, where he surprised his fiancee and upset her feminine plans for a fitting trousseau by insisting on an immediate*

marriage. Through the advice of her mother, she finally consented and they were married in the Endowment House in Salt Lake City, Utah, on August 28, 1879 by Elder Joseph F. Smith....

Shortly afterward, they started for their new home alone, but later met two families from Ogden which proved beneficial for each, as Loce knew the trail well and the others relieved the monotony of the journey.

As a means of encouragement and a source of consolation in food deficiencies, poor water, or similar conditions to be met, Loce would frequently speak of the wonderful bread and milk to be had in such abundance at the journey's end. Well, the trip ended, as all trips must do, and upon pulling into camp, they found their friends who so anxiously and impatiently awaited the coming of Loce's bride—with true hospitality had prepared a feast of the best the fort afforded. With much joy and some misgiving they were seated together at the bountiful board, and Clara, recognizing the much talked about MILK, reached for her bowl, tasted it and set it down. Later she tried again and finally said, "Well, if it comes back forever, I'll not drink that milk." Loce, wishing to save his bride an infraction of the rules, drank it for her. The strained feeling dawned at last on the hosts when a child refused to drink its milk also. Investigation then proved the milk to be in that sickly "blue–john" stage, so unpalatable to all. The trouble had arisen when a sour milk pan, instead of a sweet, had hurriedly been brought from the row of shelves in the milk-house. The event was speedily forgiven when the fresh milk, in quantity and quality which Loce had advertized so fluently, was served as needed.[18]

In the early days of the Church, people were picky too, about whether the milk was sweet or sour. But, sometimes the circumstances were such that they had to lay their fussiness aside and be grateful for what they had:

Saturday, the 17th, we camped in the township of Wayne, in Indiana; myself and many of the brethren were much fatigued and sore-footed, and our stockings wet with blood, we having traveled forty miles. I called at a house and drank the first buttermilk I ever drank in my life. I told the company what I had been drinking, when they produced a bucket and desired me to get them some. I went and got a bucket full. They all drank

> *heartily until it came to R— O—, who complained that the bucket was one which the horses drank out of. I told him if he had seen the churn he would not complain of the bucket. I need not say they drank all the buttermilk and sent for more...*[19]

This was during the time of Zion's Camp and the narrator of this story, was Apostle George A. Smith.

Another incident which took place with Elder Smith, of which he was so fondly in the habit of relating, was this:

> *On one occasion I observed Ezra Thayre... behind me. I waited for him; when he came up to me he dropped down upon the prairie, being overcome with the heat, and said he could travel no farther and was resolved to die there. I continued to urge him along for three miles to a little log cabin, where we asked for some water, and were told they had none, and that there was none nearer than three miles; we asked for milk, vinegar, or whiskey, but they had none. Ezra Thayre then said: 'Madam have you anything in the world that is wet?' She thought a moment, and then replied, 'I believe I have a little buttermilk, though my cow has not been home for three months.' She then brought out a rusty old coffee pot and poured from it about a quart of buttermilk, which was blue and as sour as vinegar; we partook of it, and it saved Ezra's life. We then walked three miles to Mr. Payne's well, and it took several hours to allay my companion's thirst."*[20]

However, the value of buttermilk is not to be underestimated nor taken too lightly. In the past, it has been the sole means of saving life when the doctors had failed:

> *Many discouraging things happened, but the worst blow was the loss of mother's health. Her children were very kind to her, and the sons-in-law did all they could for her welfare. She was taken to doctors in Salt Lake City, in Los Angeles, and in Phoenix. Each diagnosed her case differently, but all agreed that nothing could be done for her, that is, after each had treated her for sometime, and got a good fee for their services. She continued to get worse. She had lost faith in doctors, and decided if she was to live it was "up to her." She had her daughter make poultices and apply them to where the pain was most severe, and after persistance they were effective. She was in such a condition that everyone gave her up and her children were sent for. She felt she*

was better, though so weak that for days she took no nourishment, except one or two teaspoonsful of liquid a day. Finally, she asked for BUTTERMILK. That tasted so good, that she called for more, and that was her ONLY DIET FOR A LONG TIME, and it seemed to be JUST WHAT HER SYSTEM REQUIRED, for she began to GAIN STRENGTH until she was well, and for the past four years has enjoyed better health than she had for years.[21]

A study conducted once by an eminent scientist proved that a little milk with the rest of a meal, certainly made some significant difference afterwards:

Some years ago an English scientist, Dr. F.G. Hopkins, was feeding some rats with a diet composed essentially of refined foods, such as sugar, flour, etc. All the rats received the same ration and I the same diet, except that one group received in addition a very small quantity of milk, entirely too little for full sustenance. After twenty-three days each rat had gained only about 38 grams; except the rats that had received a little milk in their diet. These had gained about 88 grams each, or nearly two and one half times as much as those that had not been fed milk.

This astounding result has led to many experiments, especially by Dr. E.V. McCollum, now of Johns Hopkins University. It is now well established that there is widely distributed in plants and animals certain substances, not yet well defined, which help greatly to promote growth and physical well being. These substances are commonly known as vitamins, and are as essential to life as any other part of food.[22]

Eggs also played an important part in the Mormon diet, though not as much as milk. Yet, in a sense, they are considered of the same class as the dairy products. "Joseph Smith, the founder of the Church, said of Brigham Young, that 'he could eat more eggs, and beget more children, than any man in the State of Illinois.'"[23] It points up the fact that some made the results of a hen's strenuous efforts part of their daily routine of eating—and rather large at that, judging from what Brother Young must have been able to consume in one sitting.

Cow's milk was not the only kind consumed by Latter-day Saints. Some preferred goat milk to the other types of food:

My mind had been taxed to the utmost all this time. I had been in the farther end of a crowded lodge, with no reasonable probability of getting out of it if I wished to, and without the privilege of inhaling a breath of fresh air.

Some roasted mutton was brought in and presented to me to take the first rib.

The sight of the roast meat, the sudden change of affairs, together with the recollection of the threats of a very different roast to the one I had on hand, turned my stomach. I said to those around me, "I am sick."

I went to the door of the lodge. It was refreshing to breathe in the open air, and look out into the glorious moonlight. I thought it was midnight; if so, the council had lasted about twelve hours.

A woman's heart seems kindlier than man's among all people. A Navajo woman, seeming to comprehend my situation, came to me and asked me if she could not get me something I would like to eat.

She mentioned several varieties of food she had on hand, none of which I desired. She said she had been at my house in Kanab, and she saw I liked milk, and she would get me some. With a dish in her hand, she went about among the goats, stripping them by moonlight.

She brought me about a pint of milk, which I drank, went into the lodge and lay down and slept until some of the party said it was light enough to see to get our horses.[24]

For some, though, securing milk for themselves to drink without a vessel or container in which to put it was not all that easy:

My wife remained in the city with me during the time we were delivering the goods, some three weeks. After getting through, I, in company with W. Roberts of Provo, fitted up a team and went back to trade.

Roberts remained at the South Pass while I went down with two yoke of oxen to Devil's Gate. It may be interesting to some to give a brief description of my trip going down, some ninety miles. Stephen Markham was in charge of the Y.X. station at the South Pass. He had nine head of good milk cows which he had orders to send to Devil's Gate for the use of men stationed there. He offered to furnish me a horse if I would drive them down. This was agreeable, as I would have had to foot it otherwise.

As I could not carry provisions very well, and having money, it was supposed that I could buy bread at least, as there were trains of California emigrants continually on the road. Cups were scarce, so when I started out I had nothing but my blankets and gun. I happened to have a new clay pipe in my pocket. After asking several persons to sell me a cup and some bread and being refused, I concluded to see if I could not get through with what I had. The cows all gave plenty of milk and were gentle. I necessarily had to milk them to keep their udders from spoiling.

So when I would get a cow all milked but the strippings, I would put the stem of the pipe into my mouth and milk into the bowl and draw the milk through. This was about the same as sucking "mint julep" with a straw. I enjoyed it immensely, being fond of new milk.

I found it so much better than eating rawhide that I ceased asking the emigrants I met for either a cup or bread. I made the trip through in less than four days; probably felt a little "calfish" but never lost my flesh or strength.[25]

Daniel W. Jones' feeling of being "calfish" only seemed natural in the light of the circumstances under which he had to drink his milk. On the other hand, however, a calf, in drinking its share from a pail, could make a man feel a mite "swearish" at times:

It is told that in his younger days, before he became a high church official, J. Golden Kimball, once got all dressed up in his Sunday best to go to Church. Then he discovered that the calf hadn't been fed. So he took a bucket of skimmed milk and went out to the corral. The hungry calf lunged forward, submerged his muzzle clear up to his eyes in the milk, then raised his head and snorted, blowing foam all over J. Golden's clothes. "If I wasn't a member of the church," he shrieked, "If I wasn't an officer in the priesthood, if I wasn't trying to forswear swearing, and if I couldn't control my temper, I'd take your goddamned head and drown you in this here bucket!"[26]

No matter which way it is consumed or fed, good, whole, raw milk, as the pioneers drank, is "udderly" good for the system of man.

NOTES

1. John Henry Evans, *Joseph Smith, An American Prophet*; New York, 1946; p. 182.

2. C.V. Hansen, *Church News,* December, 1935. Also: *Juvenile Instructor,* 27:129.

3. Conference Report, 1899, p. 47.

4. Heiser, *op., cit.*, p. 101. (Previous chapter notes).

5. "Joseph The Prophet"; *The Salt Lake Herald* Supplement, Saturday, January 12, 1895; p. 210

6. Joseph Fielding Smith, *Life of Joseph F. Smith*; Salt Lake, 1938; p. 128.

7. Journal of Henry William Bigler, Church Historian's Office. Salt Lake City.

8. *Millennial Star* 93:150.

9. *DEC* 4:4.

10. *Juvenile Instructor* 27:385-386.

11. Diary of L. John Nuttall (May, 1889 - Feb. 1890) p. 543; Harold B. Lee Library, Special Collections, Brigham Young University, Provo, Utah.

12. Orson F. Whitney, *Whitney's Popular History of Utah*; p. 51.

13. *Era* 73:59 (April, 1970 issue).

14. Letter of Captain James Brown to his family, February 22, 1854, from New Orleans, Louisiana, while he was Emigration Agent for the Church; Utah Humanities Foundation Collection, University of Utah, Western Americana section, Mariott Library.

15. *Pine Valley Days*, by Julia Putnam Foster. Utah Human Foundation, University of Utah, *op., cit.*

16. *Juvenile Instructor* 33:360.

17. Heiser, *op., cit.*, p. 102.

18. "Pioneer Women—Incidents from the life of Mrs. Clara G. Rogers"; Roberta Clayton Manuscript Collection, Harold B. Lee Library, BYU; folder #142 box 3.

19. *The Contributor* 4:44.

20. *The Contributor* 4:81.

21. Annie C. H. Whipple, folder #184, box 4; Roberta Clayton, *op., cit.*

22. Young Men's Mutual Improvement Association Senior Manual 1922-23, "Health and Achievement"; p. 24.

23. Jules Remy and Julius Brenchley, *A Journey To Great Salt Lake City*; London, MDCCCLXI; p. 201.

24. James A. Little, *Jacob Hamblin—Fifth Book of The Faith-Promoting Series*; Salt Lake City, 1881; pp. 118-119.

25. Daniel W. Jones, *Forty Years Among The Indians;* Salt Lake City, 1890; p. 115.

26. Austin and Alta Fife, *Saints of Sage & Saddle*; Indiana, 1956; pp. 310—311.

CHAPTER FOUR

THE STAFF OF LIFE

(The Prophets on Whole Grain Food)

Bread is as ancient as the scriptures themselves, and as modern as the Restored Gospel is today. "By the sweat of thy face shalt thou eat bread."[1]

> *He told the churchman that he always fixed the time of hoeing his large field, to that when he could secure the services of Joseph Smith, because of the influence that boy had over the wild boys of the neighborhood, and explained that when these boys or young men worked by themselves much time would be spent in arguing and quarrelling which often ended in a ring fight. But when Joseph Smith worked with them, the work went steadily forward and he got the full worth of the wages he paid.*[2]

The sharing of this substance with one's fellowman is as old as history, and as recent as modern times. "Bring me, I pray thee, a morsel of bread in thine hand."[3]

> *Brother B. Young further said, relative to a certain difficulty arising out of a circumstance concerning some bread that brother J.S. Carter, on their journey to Missouri on the line between Ohio and Indiana, said to Brother Joseph, "Is this thing right?" "What thing?" Concerning Parley P. Pratt asking brother Sylvester Smith for some bread for supper? He then learned that brother Pratt had asked brother Sylvester for some bread; that brother Sylvester had bread at the time, but directed him to someone else who he (brother S.) said had a sufficient (amount); that brother Pratt called upon that individual and could not obtain any. That he was present when brother Joseph told brother Sylvester that he had not conducted himself right in the matter. That he ought to impart what he had in preference to directing one where he was not certain he could obtain; that by so doing some might be deprived of food at times. He further said*

> *that brother S. contended he had been right and justified his own conduct in the matter. That brother Joseph entreated with brother Sylvester to convince him; that he, brother S. was in a fault, but he continued to justify his course till brother J. reproved him sharply...*
>
> *Brother Lyman Sherman said that he concurred in brother B. Young's statements concerning the bread. That he thought it was generally known that brother Pratt, in consequence of brother Sylvester not furnishing him with bread, was deprived of bread that night...*[4]

Since the beginning of time, men have grumbled at things, and complained about the bread they had. "And the people spake against God...our soul loatheth this light bread."[5]

> *One time in Nauvoo, some English brethren did not like to eat corn bread, and one of them says to another, just before partaking of some, "Are you going to ask a blessing? I am not going to thank God for nothing else but corn bread..."*[6]

The Lord has made use of grain in a symbolic sense, in visions of the night. "And Joseph dreamed a dream, and he told it to his brethren...behold, we were binding sheaves in the field, and lo, my sheaf arose, and also stood upright; and, behold, your sheaves stood round about, and made obeisance to my sheaf."[7]

> *October 25, 1857, Sunday... (in Hawaii)... I am reminded of a dream I had a few nights ago. I dreamed I was in a chamber room of some old house and on the floor were several piles of wheat. Some large and some small and the smallest pile of wheat was the cleanest and in the same situation it was where it was put there. But the other piles were leveled nearly to the floor and the grain scattered more or less all over the floor and was very dirty for I thought the rats, mice and cats had been all over and in it and I could see their very tracks and I commenced to push the wheat together and to sweep it up and when I began to examine it closely, I found that the cats had made the biggest pile of wheat their necessary and deposit of filth for I found rolls of it in the wheat. What I done with the wheat I do not remember. But from what I see and learn from the Utah Elders now on the Islands, there are only a few native Saints here and they are the ones living on the Island of Lanai, the gathering place, where I may say is the smallest pile of wheat and the*

cleanest.

Corn and wheat are both considered to be members of the grain family. As such, both have been used in parables, comparing things prophetic and philosophical with the reality around us. "For, lo, I will command, and I will sift the house of Israel among all nations, like as corn is sifted in a sieve, yet shall not the least grain fall upon the earth."[9]

Shortly before his martyrdom, the Prophet attended a meeting at Nauvoo.

> *Before the meeting opened he was sitting with head bowed as if in deep thought. A brother named Cutler laid a hand heavily upon his shoulder and said, "Brother Joseph, raise your head." Then brother Cutler reminded the Prophet of all his power and greatness saying many words of praise to him, and ended by telling him to face the world with head erect.*
>
> *The Prophet referred brother Cutler to a field of ripened grain, saying that the heads that bow low upon their stalks are filled with ripened grain ready for the gleaner's gathering, while those heads that stand erect upon their stalks have no fulness in them for the Master's storehouse and must be gathered with the straw.*[10]

In times of dire circumstances, sometimes any kind of bread would do. "Thou feedest them with the bread of tears."[11]

> *"When Brother Brigham left home...all his family had was one barrel of rotten flour."*[12]

* * *

> *"Of all the unpleasant memories, not one half so bitter as that dreary six months' voyage in an emigrant ship...but we trusted in God and he heard our prayers; and when I soaked the mouldy ship bread...and fried it in the tallow...God made it sweet to me and to my child, for on this food I weaned her. I used to think of Hagar and her babe, and of the God who watched over them, and again I remembered the voice and the words it spoke unto me—and took courage.*[13]

When there is great suffering in the land, even the little ones learn to appreciate something so simple as a little flour. "The young children ask bread, and no man breaketh it unto them."[14]

...starvation was our fate. For we was reduced to 4 ounces of flour a day for all those who were over 12 years of age, and 2 ounces for those under that age and nothing else.... Then was the time to hear children crying for something to eat; just a little bread please. Nearly all the children would cry themselves to sleep every night. My 2 little brothers would get the sack that had flour in and turn it long side out and suck and lick the flour dust off it.[15]

Among the people of God, both ancient and modern, there were those who used the benefits of grain to their own selfish end and good advantage. "They are they who eat up my people. They eat bread and call not upon the Lord."[16]

Peter Haws sworn. Said that he came to Nauvoo before the Laws and brought considerable property. It was a short time after the Church had been driven out of Missouri, and were in a starving condition. By the counsel of the Presidency, witness converted his funds to feeding the poor, bringing in meat and flour, and corn; and while thus engaged, drew upon the Laws, who were at that time engaged in merchandise, to the amount of some six hundred dollars, which, on account of expenditure for the poor, he was not able to pay within seventy or eighty dollars, which they pressed him for as soon as they wanted it, although he offered them good property at considerable less than the market value, as witness was obliged to leave the city on Church business for a little season. William Law threatened and intimidated witness' family during his absence for the pay.

Dr. Foster made a public dinner on the 4th day of July. Witness was obliged to be absent, and deposited meat, flour, and corn, with William Law to give to the poor at the dinner, and Law handed it out as his own private property. Witness carried a load of wheat to Law's mill to be ground. Law would not grind it only to give a certain quantity of flour in return by weight. Law used up the flour, promising from time to time he would refund it. As witness was about to start on a mission to the south with his valise in his hand, saw Law before his door talking with Hyrum Smith. Called on Law, and told him he was going away, and his family wanted the flour. Law promised on the honor of a gentleman and a Saint, that his family should have the flour when they wanted...

Hawes said when he returned he found his family must

have starved, if they had not borrowed money to get food somewhere else; could not get it of Law; and Law was preaching punctuality, punctuality, punctuality, as the whole drift of his discourses to the Saints, and abusing them himself and grinding the poor.[17]

A man's own family could be found in such straits that it would be necessary for them to obtain grain foodstuff from just about any source possible. "I seen...his seed begging bread."[18]

One day we had been without flour for so long and no bread to eat, Mother and I were walking down one of the streets in Salt Lake City and we saw a piece of bread lying on the ground. Mother would have passed it by but I cried so hard for it she let me pick it up and eat it and never in my life have I ever tasted anything so good to me as that piece of bread did.[19]

One's appetite may be content with just a slice of grain product. "Thou shalt be satisfied with bread."[20] On the other hand, if the diet has been without it for considerable time, it may take some readjusting of the system to get used to wheat:

At this time we were well recruited, having had plenty of meat for some time, but scarcely any flour for some five months. Bread we had hardly tasted. In fact, the first biscuit I got almost choked me; I had entirely lost my appetite for it.[21]

In the teachings of Jesus Christ is found the principle that "whatsoever a man measureth out, the same shall be measured back unto him again." "Cast thy bread upon the waters; for thou shalt find it after many days."[22]

Friday, January 21, 1881. At night went to the prayer meeting at Father Perkins. Father McBride spoke in a very edifying manner...

Spoke of the marvelous manner the Lord had put flour into his barrel in the times of famine and distress in the early settlement of these mountain valleys, and that he had always divided his scanty portion agreeable to the wishes of his Bishop and always found enough put in the barrel to use for days until wheat was ready and then the usual supply ceased to be found as before.[23]

In the face of hardship, the difficulty under which bread might have to be made could be most severe. "The Lord give you the bread of affliction."[24]

> *Sunday, December 20, 1846. This morning we arose very early and brother Green came with some water, thick with mud, which he succeeded in getting by going two miles. With this we mixed some bread. It looked very black. We also made some gravy but it took but very little flour. It was so thick with mud, it resembled clay mortar very much and tasted very strong of the same. Just as we were through eating our muddy repast, the bugle was blown for a march....*[25]

Charity is an understood thing of the heart. It is something God expects us to show. "Is it not to deal thy bread to the hungry?"[26] Should we decline such acts of service to our fellow-man, the resulting action may prove fatal.

> *"June 26, 1835. On our way we called at several places for dinner and were refused. At the home of Mr. Thatcher, near Andover corners, on asking for refreshment, they declared they had no bread and nothing cooked in the house, and were too busy to bake bread for us. They afterwards reported that they had plenty of bread, but they would not give it to the Mormons. About six weeks after this we preached in that neighborhood, and on passing by the house in company with Mr. Frederick Pendleton, who had heard them tell the circumstance of turning the Mormon preachers away empty, when they had bread enough, he exclaimed to a bystander: "Thatcher's folks turned away the boys with the excuse that they had no bread when they had plenty, and God Almighty has sent a frost and destroyed all their corn, so they'll have no bread next year, sure enough!" (We being so young were known to that country by the name of the 'Mormon boys'.) The fact was that a streak of frost, about a quarter of a mile wide, had completely killed all the corn and other grain on Thatcher's farm, leaving the rest of the neighborhood untouched."*[27]

And then there are the undeserving, whose claim on bread for survival is no more legitimate than Lucifer's is for salvation. "They eat the bread of wickedness."[28] "As for myself," Brigham Young said, "I would rather the grasshoppers would eat the wheat than the cursed Gentiles!"[29]

Where the righteous may stand on the brink of extinction

through lack of adequate supplies, the Lord can, somehow, provide a remedy for their needs. "I will satisfy her poor with bread."[30] Throughout the winter of 1848-9, food was scarce among the Mormon settlers... Wheat had ranged from $4 to $5...a bushel...the small quantity of breadstuffs that remained, were however, distributed among the poor in such quantities as to prevent actual starvation.[31]

The "staff of life" could also be the "staff of friendship," and had a peculiar way of bringing people together more often. "Mine own familiar friend, in whom I trusted, did eat of my bread."[32]

> *It was through Mother's influence that we as a family held a Family Hour by lamplight each morning, where she read from the Scriptures and we sang a song and had prayer before breakfast, while the whole-wheat cereal was cooking on the wood stove. (Circa 1880's1890's).*[33]

Anticipating journeys of considerable length, ancient Israel generally met such occasions with plenty of provisions. "Moreover they that were nigh them, even unto Issachar and Zebulun and Naphtali, brought bread on asses, and on camels, and on mules, and on oxen, and meat, meal, cakes of figs and bunches of raisins, and wine, and oil...abundantly."[34] In modern times, similar preparations have been made when gathering Israel from the four quarters of the earth:

> *Tuesday and Thursday following most of us were very much out of sorts through sea sickness, but some of us escaped without any sickness. During these days our dear president, Captain Dan Jones, was very mindful of the sick. He showed his love towards us very much as he would walk back and forth through the great ship, and administer to those that were sick.*
>
> *He and Brother David Daniels of Brechfa and William Jenkins of Cardiff and other faithful ones were very busy waiting on us and making gruel for those that were sick. This was the most tasty and beneficial food for us during these days. It would stay on the stomach better than anything else. I did not want either salt or butter with the gruel, nor could I eat any bread with it. It was the same with my dear wife and children. But Mary, my youngest daughter, was not sick during the whole voyage, though many prophesied before we left Wales that this one would surely die on the sea, because she was nursing her mother; but to our Heavenly Father be the glory for keeping us all alive. We did not remain sick but a few days, and I see by this*

time that the sea sickness has done us good by purifying our stomachs. I recommend all those that will follow us to Zion to bring OAT MEAL AND OAT BREAD with them—they will find this the best food when they are sea sick.[35]

What is generally thought of as the main staple to satisfy hunger can also have other purposes as well, besides filling the human body with something good. "It is written, Man shall not live by bread alone."[36] Even the food grains, primarily classed among the "meats to maintain life," were drafted into medical use—mainly as external applications. Wheat was deemed a cure for wounds, and white bread poultices then, as now, were applied to sties. Oats also made popular poultices—one for impetigo and one for a "stitch in the side." Gerard adds waspishly: "Otemeale is good for to make a faire and well coloured maide to looke like a cake of tallow, especially if she take next her stomacke a good draft of strong vinegar after it." Rye was a specific for abscesses, while millet meal mixed with tar made a dressing for snake bite.[37]

* * *

A thick, old-fashioned, oatmeal mush was the basis for a mustard plaster. In cases of croup, or pneumonia, where there was congestion, oil, lard, or sweet cream was rubbed on the skin to keep it from blistering. One level tablespoonful of mustard was stirred into the mush, then it was put in a bag and flattened into a plaster. A layer or two of cloth was put on first, such as a piece of old sheeting, then the hot plaster was laid on, and covered with another layer of cloth. This was left on for two hours and when it was taken off, great care was used to keep the patient from being fanned with cold air. Layers of warm cloth were left on all night, or until the sick one was to be sponged off, to remove the perspiration, which was usually profuse...

My father's youngest sister, Sarah Emma Kartchner Miller, gave us two remedies which she said were excellent for congestion of the lungs. One was a MUSH MADE OF CORN MEAL stirred into boiling vinegar. Sprinkle cayenne pepper into the mush, then proceed as with other packs.[38]

White bread is comfortable to the senses. It is smooth to the taste, and appealing to the pampered Nature of modern man. It is soft and requires minimal effort in chewing. Yet the characteristics of its refinement are not new to twentieth-century technology. In another time, in another Babylon, such things existed too. However, the Prophet of God alive then abstained from this "civilized" food for ascetic reasons. "In those days, I Daniel...ate no pleasant bread."[39]

"...store bread as turned out by our big commercial bakeries is no better eating nowadays. Instead of rich, crunchy, satisfying crust, it has a thin, tasteless, flabby coating. True, the stuff is now wrapped in wax paper. It comes ready-sliced and is 'enriched' with synthetic vitamins—which costs little and makes good ballyhoo.

"Millions of dollars are spent in shrieking its alleged virtues over the radio, plastering the landscape with billboard advertising. It is, undoubtedly, pure, sanitary, wholesome, nutritious, clean, white, and beautiful—but it is UTTERLY TASTELESS...

"This is not just my opinion. There is a good deal of evidence to show that the general public doesn't like the big baker's product either. We buy it—but our national taste has not become so debased that we have grown fond of the guilt stuffing foisted upon us as the staff of life."[40]

Having worked in the restaurant business for several years, the author has found that whenever rolls, pies, or other baked goods were advertised as "home made," that is, made by the establishments themselves, people seemed to prefer them over the regular variety commonly found in large-scale bakeries and supermarkets everywhere these days. One dining house, in particular, which took pride in serving "the real thing," did a brisk business in customer trade, while some of its competitors down the road barely managed.

"The sad fact is that the great majority of Americans fill their bellies with store bread not because they like it but because it is difficult for them to get anything else."[41]

Another great Man of God like unto Daniel, President Heber C. Kimball, advised the Latter-day Saints: "FINE FLOUR IS NOT GOOD. The finer the flour we eat, THE SHORTER WILL BE OUR LIVES. It would be better for us to eat coarse bread, such as the Graham bread."[42]

But there are those in our midst even today who would continue to advocate the use of the other, despite this noble man's stern warning.

Enriched white flour has almost as much iron as does whole wheat. The iron is in a form that is readily used by the body. Thiamin, riboflavin, and niacin are three B vitamins added. Enriched flour has twice as much riboflavin as the average in whole wheat. The thiamin content is almost the same in the two flours, and whole-wheat has about one fifth more niacin than is added to enriched flour.[43]

Concerning such men of reputed "knowledge," the Apostle Paul said: "Take heed therefore, unto yourselves...for I know this, that after my departing shall grievous wolves enter in among you, not sparing the flock."[44] Heber C. Kimball is no longer with us, but his words still remain. They are eternal words of life and truth. Can we afford to ignore them?

President Brigham Young said:

There is no doubt whatever that the food we eat—which is absolutely necessary to sustain us—contains poison. I do not dispute that the poison contained in the bread that has been distributed from the table this afternoon, if extracted by a skillful chemist, would be enough to kill. Where we find so much poison in articles the people will become very strongly attached to them in a very short time.[45]

Yet the sophist intellect of modern schools would try to tell us otherwise:

There is no experimental proof that the eating of white bread is injurious to the humans. White flour is not poisonous... Contrary also to reports of uninformed persons, poisonous substances are not added to wheat at commercial mills to prevent spoilage nor to bleach flour... Bleached flour is not harmful as many people are led to believe... Housewives can make better quality bread and other baked products with bleached than unbleached flour.[46]

Well did the Saviour say, when he predicted: "...beware of false prophets, who come to you in sheep's clothing; but inwardly they are ravening wolves."[47] All of the scientific jargon and fancy talk in our society will not be able to replace the inspired words of great men. No matter whether certain kinds of bread can "help build strong bodies 12 ways," there is *NO WAY* that such crass commercialism can ever justify a cheap product in light of what the Prophets have said.

Brigham Young and Heber C. Kimball spoke by the Spirit of the Living God when they uttered these words of sensible nutrition, and their fine counsel still cries from the dust to those who will hear and believe in their report.

> *"White bread is made of flour which has been robbed of its most valuable parts, the bran and the germ; for therein are found the mineral and the precious vitamin B. The body needs ALL of the grain for food. The sisters should use whole-wheat in all their baking in place of white flour. The Word says, 'wheat for man—not a part of the kernel only.'"*[48]

Brigham Young advised mothers in Israel to give their children bread—"not soft bread; teach your children to eat crust—hard baked bread...."[49] The hard bread, of which he was speaking, is what we would call the "stale" kind. However, such simple fare seems to have suited the pioneers just fine:

> *When I first sat down on this ground, in 1847, I was dressed in buckskin, having torn most of my clothes to pieces. I had rawhide soles on my feet, and had A PIECE OF HARD BREAD and a piece of dried antelope meat to eat.*[50]

The man speaking was none other than Apostle George A. Smith, and he certainly seems to have enjoyed his repast, according to the lively manner of expression found in his delivery that day.

The Widstoes, John and Leora, had many good things to say about the use of wheat flour in preference to white flour. The Apostle of the Lord had these remarks to make in connection with it:

> *There are at least five social, economic considerations which have delayed the general acceptance of the verdict of science. First, white flour may be kept indefinitely, while whole wheat flour must be used within rather narrow limits of time... Second, there are large milling interests which protect their investments by vigorous advertising... Third, there is a foolish prejudice on the part of many persons against the color of whole wheat bread. The whiter the flour, the better they like it. To meet this prejudice chemicals are often used to bleach the flour to a dead white color... Fourth, people who have eaten white bread all their lives are accustomed to the taste, and require some time to learn to enjoy the nutty, sweet taste of whole wheat bread. Fifth, the incorrect notion has been fostered that whole wheat bread*

injures the stomach. Long experience has shown the fallacy of such a belief, if the stomach is normal. By proper grinding, the whole wheat flour may be made as fine as white flour. For weaker stomachs, flour made from wheat with the extreme outer covering of the kernel removed, could be used.

All these objections, pitted against man's need of health, are valueless and fall to the ground.

It is because of the structure of the wheat berry that whole wheat bread is better than white bread...

Chemical analyses agree that there is no question about the superiority of whole wheat bread over white bread.

Cases of improved health have frequently been reported when the diet has been changed only from white to whole wheat bread...Much disease is caused by an unbalanced diet, in which white bread forms a large part.

The evidence for whole wheat flour, as against white refined flour in human nutrition, is complete and unanswerable. It is a reflection of the contrariness of human Nature, when millers report surpluses, as they do today, of the better parts of the wheat, and are compelled to sell them at lower prices because of a false conception of food values. It is even less pardonable when people, knowing the truth, will not observe it, because of tradition or appetite. People who bring disease upon themselves, by ignoring truth, deserve LITTLE SYMPATHY!

There are those who say that what white flour lacks they will supply by eating other foods very rich in the missing substances. That sounds plausible, but is seldom attained. Poorer people cannot always afford to buy the necessary supplements. Richer people often forget, in the face of appetite, what should be done. It is best to eat all of our foods much as Nature offers them...

The spirit of the Word of Wisdom is that we shall seek good physical health by abstinence from harmful things, and by the proper selection of our foods, so that great blessings, physical, mental, and spiritual, may follow. "All grain is ordained for the use of man—to be the staff of life." So the positive aspects of this divine law of health declare; and they should be used in accordance with our present understanding of the composition of grains. THERE IS NO REASON FOR ASSUMING THAT THE LORD MEANT A PART OF THE GRAIN KERNEL. The regular use of whole wheat bread and cereal would greatly increase our health and protect us against disease.[51]

And upon the same matter, his wife said:

Well may bread and cereals be called "the Staff of Life," for they form the large proportion of the food for most of the peoples on the earth. The less there is for food in the family budget the more largely are grain products used for the family food; for they are economical in price and are nutritious in content. Grain products, to be nutritious, should be prepared with their FULL FOOD CONTENT, not devitalized and refined, as is so often done to satisfy an artificial demand for dead white foods or for commercial purposes.

There is no excuse for using white bread. In nutritive quality it is so much inferior to the whole grain product that one who would be well should never tolerate it. Not only is the whole grain far richer in mineral and vitamin content, but "the proteins of white flour are much less valuable in nutrition than are the proteins of the whole wheat."

Does it not seem more than unwise to persist in eating devitalized food just to cater to a perverted appetite? When it is well established that certain foods are needed by the body for full nourishment, one should have the gumption to learn to like them—to re-educate the taste if necessary. By the same token is it not foolish to make bread with only part whole wheat flour? If a food is best for one, it should be used—no compromise—no "half and half" may take the place of the genuine article.[52]

President Brigham Young said:

I have many and many a time said to children when they begged for the soft bread... "Look here; you will not live very long; you will probably come to a premature grave." I have noticed invariably the child that selects the soft bread to be a short-lived person. The children that hunt around after the crust, and eat it, I have noticed endure, live, and continue to live on.[53]

From the Prophets, we have learned the following about refined bread:

(a) they themselves avoided it (Daniel).

(b) they said it was no good (Heber C. Kimball).

(c) they said it would *SHORTEN ONE'S LIFE SPAN CONSIDERABLY* (Brigham and Heber).

(d) refined bread contains poisons (Brigham Young).

(e) they recommended the use of graham bread (Heber) and hard bread (Brigham), in place of the other.

(f) it is foolish to use white flour; and those who do so, deserve *VERY LITTLE SYMPATHY* when they get sick later on (Apostle John A. Widstoe).

Still, in the light of all this evidence from on High, there will be many who will continue to ignore the Servants of God, and proceed their own careless ways down the paths of misguided concepts, false traditions, unjustified prejudice, and in the end, ill health as a final, climactic result for their silly behavior.

Perhaps the most noble tribute which can be given "the staff of life," is in an emblematic sense of deep reverence. Jesus said, "I am the bread of life."[54]

> *Every Sunday the Sacrament is administered; the tables loaded with the baskets of bread and silver tankards of water... occupying a dais at the foot of the pulpits, upon which several bishops take their places, and break the bread into fragments. Precisely at two o'clock the great organ sends forth its melodious invocation, and the subdued noise of neighborly gossip, which, as the Madame said, "seemed the veritable humming of the honey bees of Deseret in their house hive," is wholly hushed. The music at the Tabernacle is far-famed in the west, and gives constant delight to all the people. The singing is followed by a long prayer by some one of the dignitaries in or about the pulpits, during which the time is utilized to prepare the bread and water; and as soon as the prayer has ceased a large number of brethren begin to pass the sacred food and drink.*
>
> *Everybody, old and young, partakes, and it is an hour and a half before the communion is completed. Meanwhile someone of the highest officers of the Church, or perhaps two or three of them in succession, has been preaching; so that two long*

> *hours are exhausted before dismissal. Such was the experience of our visit, and it was an average occasion.*[55]

Such was how a typical Sabbath went in the year 1884 on Temple Square. But one can certainly be assured that "the whole kernel" was used, and not a part of it. Or, in other words, they used *GOOD, WHOLE WHEAT BREAD* for the tokens in remembrance. After all, it is best to give the Lord something *WHOLE,* instead of something *HALF. WHITE BREAD IS A "BROKEN STAFF." AVOID IT.*[56]

For, as the Scriptures say, it is the "bread of deceit."[57]

NOTES

1. Genesis 3:25 (*Joseph Smith's Inspired Version of the Bible*).

2. Lafayette C. Lee, "*Reminiscences of Joseph Smith*"; handwritten ms., BYU.

3. I Kings 17:11.

4. Kirtland High Council Minutes, August 29, 1834; Church Historian's Office, SLC; being the High Council trial of Sylvester Smith, for alleged misconduct and inappropriate behavior not becoming a Latter-day Saint, while engaged with the rest of his brethren in the Zion's Camp maneuvers of some time earlier.

5. Numbers 21:5.

6. *JD* 3:11.

7. Genesis 37:5—6.

8. *Journal of Henry William Bigler*, Church Historian's Office, Salt Lake City.

9. Amos 9:9.

10. Lafayette C. Lee ms., *op., cit.* See also *Juvenile Instructor* 27:203, for another version of this, in published form. However, in its edited state, the Elder's name was omitted, and the context more briefly shortened. However, an additional paragraph appended to the printed one, indicates that the unnamed Elder (Brother Cutler) later apostatized and went back East.

11. Psalms 80:5.

12. *JD* 18:124.

13. Augusta Joyce Crocheron, *Representative Women of Deseret*; Salt Lake, 1884; pp. 101—102.

14. Lamentations 4:4.

15. Journal of Heber McBride, p. 19; Harold B. Lee Library, Special Collections, Brigham Young University, Provo, Utah. This incident took place in the winter of 1856, during the fatal Martin Handcart Company disaster.

16. Psalms 14:4.

17. DHC 6:440—441.

18. Psalms 37:25.

19. DUP Huntington Chapter History, "History of Elizabeth Hill Johnson," fd. 2, item #29; Harold B. Lee Library, Special Collections, BYU, Provo, Utah.

20. Proverbs 20:13.

21. Daniel W. Jones, *op., cit.*, p. 102 (previous chapter notes).

22. Ecclesiastes 11:1.

23. Diary of Charles L. Walker, p. 670; Harold B. Lee Library, BYU, Provo.

24. Isaiah 30:20.

25. William E. King Journals (1837-1847). Church Historian's Office, Salt Lake.

26. Isaiah 58:7.

27. *The Contributor* 4:83.

28. Proverbs 4:17.

29. Journal of Jacob Hamblin, p. 20.

30. Psalms 132:15.

31. Bancroft, *op., cit.*, p. 288. (Previous chapter notes).

32. Psalms 41:9.

33. Sarah Roundy Berry; Roberta Clayton Collection, *op., cit.*, folder #5, bx 1.

34. I Chronicles 12:40.

35. Kate B. Carter, Historical Pamphlet, December, 1943, pp. 39–391.

36. Matthew 4:4.

37. *Natural History* Magazine, December, 1959; "The Roots of Healing—Ancient Herbals"; pp. 587-588.

38. DUP Lesson for October, 1957, "And They Were Healed"; pp. 107-108. Compiled by Kate B. Carter.

39. Daniel 10:2—3.

40. Clarence Woodbury, "Our Daily Bread"; The Reader's Digest, May, 1945, p. 49.

41. *Ibid.*

42. *JD* 12:191.

43. "Facts About Foods and Nutrition," Utah State Agricultural College Extension Bulletin, No. 266, May 1953.

44. Acts 20 28—29

45. *JD* 13:276.

46 "Health Aspects of The Word of Wisdom" by David D. Geddes. Delivered during the 33rd Annual Leadership Week at Brigham Young University, with the theme "Widening Horizons"; p. 17.

47. Matthew 7:24 (Inspired Version).

48. *Millennial Star* 93:150.

49. *JD* 19:67.

50. *JD* 13:121.

51. *The Improvement Era*, December, 1945, pp. 742-744.

52. Leah Widstoe, *op., cit.*, pp. 151-152. (Cited in previous chapter notes).

53. *JD* 19:68.

54. John 6:48.

55. Ernest Ingersoll, *The Crest of The Continent*; Chicago, 1885; p. 327.

56. *Millennial Star* "Word of Wisdom" Supplement, Volume 93, p. 3.

57. Proverbs 20:17.

CHAPTER FIVE

FROM THE FRUIT OF THE VINE

(Joseph Smith and Pure Concord Grape Wine)

Brigham Young once said:

> *It is the fashion in the world to embrace men in their faith, or a fine meeting house, or a genteel congregation, thinking, "O, what perfect order, and how pretty they look; how straight they walk to meeting, and how long their faces are during the services; how pretty that deacon looks under the pulpit; the people are so pretty, the meeting house is so nice, that we want to join such pretty people." Such feelings will take a people to hell. Embrace a doctrine that will purge sin and iniquity from your hearts, and sanctify you before God, and you are right, no matter how others act.* [1]

Or, in other words, what Brother Brigham was trying to tell us is this: "*I NEVER EMBRACE ANY MAN IN MY FAITH, ONLY THE DOCTRINE HE TEACHES.*"[2] He made this statement shortly after being informed that the Mormon Prophet, Joseph Smith, whom he had never met up to that time, drank and did a lot of other bad things, too. Now, we know for a fact that Joseph Smith led a very moral, virtuous and upright life. The Lord would never have used him for the great work which He did, had it not been so otherwise. The work of God requires "clean hands and a pure heart." Mrs. Palmer, a Gentile lady whose folks were neighbors to the Smiths when they resided at Palmyra, New York, testified to a group of Latter-day Saints in Utah, during a visit she made later on in advanced years, that in her early life, as a young child, she personally knew the great Mormon leader. And of his character and bearing in youth, she solemnly declared, "There was never *A TRUER, PURER, NOBLER BOY THAN HE...*"[3] There is no record or evidence to indicate that she ever joined the Church, but until her dying day this respectable lady never changed her views nor denied her testimony of this man of God.

These are facts which will always stand, no matter what the slander or ill report may be concerning him.

Yet there is another fact which must be considered in the light of this book, and more particularly this chapter, and that is that Joseph Smith drank wine occasionally. This is not to infer, however, that he was a winebibber, or intoxicated, as his enemies make him out to be and appear. Far from this, he was a temperate sort of man, sober in his judgment and moderate in his habits. But the necessity of having to state this fact is important to the material we must examine in order to determine to what extent the Mormon people used natural foods in their daily diet. Hence, it is for scholarly purposes that this statement is made, rather than for ambiguous ones.

It would do well to state from the outset of the matter that "wine" is "fermented juice of grapes."[4] And, inasmuch as grapes are a natural fruit of the earth, the study of their use in Mormon culture is most interesting, and makes fascinating reading as the story unfolds.

The opening quote of Brigham Young's was given to show that no matter what weaknesses the Prophet may have had, or unusual things which he did that do not seem entirely right to our way of thinking, yet *HIS TEACHINGS ARE CORRECT!*

"THE DOCTRINE HE HAS PRODUCED WILL SAVE YOU AND ME, AND THE WHOLE WORLD!"[5] So said President Young, who knew him better than most men alive then. With this in mind, the reader should realize that the subject being examined in no way deters from this noble man's greatness, nor detracts from his living memory at all. It should not shake the faith of a person to know that Joseph Smith drank wine, for Jesus did also. And if one is going to have his faith shaken in something like this, then he might as well have it tried in the Saviour's as well.

The reason for so many necessary precautions before we undertake to explore the matter at length, is simply because there are those within our faith who take such a dim view of things in light of what the Word of Wisdom says, that for them to know their beloved Prophet drank a little "fruit of the vine," could, perhaps, make a shambles of their faith and a shipwreck of their testimony. After all, it must be kept in mind what was cited earlier in this book, under the first chapter concerning herbal drinks. Did not Brother George A. Smith relate an incident which transpired at the home of the Prophet in Kirtland, Ohio, wherein a good Mormon family completely apostatized after Joseph's wife, Emma, asked them if they'd like a little tea? Now, this was after the Word of Wisdom had been given, and yet so narrow was their thinking, so straight-laced was their religion, that it fairly constricted them, cutting off all spiritual circulation and common sense as well. If such a thing happened then, who can venture to say it would not take place again in our own century? For this reason, and this alone, is such a lengthy explanation necessary, that those who would cry "dirty shame" at a naked Rennaisance statue keep in mind that the nude bust was created as a work of art to begin with, and not a piece of trashy pornography, as they would be inclined to think it was.

Wine is as old as the Testaments are, and flavors scripture with its warm accounts and stirring memories. Brigham Young offers a reason as to why the Jews drank wine:

> *...in the days of ancient Israel, while in the land of Palestine they were not blessed so profusely as we are with the crystal streams from the mountains. They were in the habit of drinking a great deal of wine, and among the few who have continued to inhabit that land, this habit I believe has been kept up to the present time. It is a wine country.*[6]

A noted Bible scholar, Dean F. W. Farrar, commented upon the type of wine these people used:

> *It has been disputed whether the Hebrew wine was fermented; but the impression produced on the mind by a general review of the above notices is that the Hebrew words indicating wine refer to fermented, intoxicating wine.*
>
> *The simple wines of antiquity were incomparably less deadly than the stupefying and ardent beverages of our western nations. The wines of antiquity were more like syrups; many of them were not intoxicant; many more intoxicant in a small degree; and all of them, as a rule, taken only when largely diluted with water. They contained, even undiluted, but 4 to 5 percent of alcohol.*[7]

Further proof of this may be found in the scriptures themselves. God's people anciently, as well as modernly, were governed by a code of health similar to our Word of Wisdom. Everyone is familiar with the present injunction, "strong drinks are not for the belly."[8] Well, listen to what He had to say to the priests of old, who ministered before Him in the Tabernacle in the wilderness:

And the Lord spake unto Aaron, saying,

DO NOT DRINK WINE NOR STRONG DRINK, thou, nor thy sons with thee, when ye go into the tabernacle of the congregation, LEST YE DIE; it shall be a statute for ever throughout your generations; And that ye may put difference between HOLY and unholy, and between unclean and clean. [9]

Here we find the Lord telling His own people (at least those who officiated in holy things) to *ABSTAIN* from spiritous beverages which might lead to intoxication. And, if they failed to heed this, then they were *TO DIE*!

Furthermore, we read again in another section of an angel instructing a woman named Manoah to keep herself pure and holy so that a choice son of God might come through her womb. This great spirit was none other than the figure Samson, and his mother was duly informed of this, in the following manner: "Now, therefore, beware, I pray thee, and *DRINK NOT WINE NOR STRONG DRINK.*"

Thus, we can see from the evidence before us that the Almighty has ever been consistent in His policies. Unlike what some would think, He has not winked at the tipsy doings of one people, and been as strict as a schoolmaster with another. No, He has always been the same, and will never change in this regard. Yet, what of the wine in Mormon diet? Did our forefathers merit some special consideration in this that we do not, or is there a more logical explanation for the use of fermented grape juice by the early converts?

The first use of wine in the history of the Mormon people seems to have been for sacramental purposes. And this came by way of commandment from God, as part of the procedure to be followed in the organization of the Church of Jesus Christ of Latter-day Saints, April 6, 1830, at the house of Peter Whitmer, Fayette, Seneca County, New York:

We then took bread, blessed it, and brake it with them; also, WINE, blessed it, and drank it with them.[11]

After this, it appears that wine became a common item to be used in the emblems of sacrifice.

Its use continued throughout most of the summer until the early part of August, 1830. A confirmation meeting had been scheduled to be held in the humble hut back of the Hale tavern. This was Emma Smith's folks' residence, and it had been agreed upon to have some newly-baptized converts meet here for that purpose. It had been the custom in the Church at that time to have the Sacrament whenever such special occasions as these arose. Since Joseph had no wine in the house, he set out to purchase some from a neighbor nearby. As he was crossing through an orchard close by, a heavenly messenger suddenly appeared in transcendent glory, and stood before him in the air. The young Prophet was somewhat taken aback by this unexpected visitation, but quickly learned the reason for the angel's presence there. It was explained to him that it was not necessary to use wine for sacramental purposes, "if it so be that ye do it with an eye single to my glory."[12]

Now, the Lord knew the hearts of the citizens in those regions. And He was definitely aware of the many enemies in those parts who might have added a little poison to any wine His Servant may have purchased from them. They were full of evil and filled with the devil, and would not hesitate to commit such wicked acts at the expense of the innocent and trusting. Therefore, He warned Joseph thusly:

> *Wherefore, a commandment I give unto you, that you shall not purchase wine neither strong drink of your enemies;*
>
> *Wherefore, you shall partake of none except it is made NEW AMONG YOU; yea, in this my Father's kingdom which shall be built up on the earth.*[13]

Returning home, the Prophet meditated upon what had been told him. Yet he and his associates had never seen water used for sacramental purposes and were reluctant to substitute it in this service. So they went ahead and "prepared" wine of their own make for this meeting, perhaps picking some green grapes and crushing the sour juice from them.[14]

Thereafter, wine made by the Saints themselves was used instead of the other:

> *My husband (Newel K. Whitney) had a very fine orchard and garden (at Kirtland); all planned and arranged according to our own taste and skill. Among other fruits we had a very great quantity of red currants, from which we had ourselves manufactured wine of a very superior flavor and quality, although purely domestic, or home-made. This wine we had appropriate for the sacrament, and was the first wine used by our people for that purpose.*[15]

Often, remarkable manifestations of great power were evidenced in these special meetings:

> *I then blessed the bread and wine, and distributed a portion to each. Many of the brethren saw a heavenly vision of the Savior, and concourses of angels, and many other things, of which each one has a record of what he saw.*[16]

Some were not so fortunate as others, though, in beholding the glories above:

> *"We partook of consecrated bread and wine, and tarried all night still waiting upon the Lord, and rejoicing in him. Some testified of having the vision of heaven opened to their view, others enjoyed the spirit of prophecy, and prophesied of many great and glorious things which were yet in the future, all of which have not yet come to pass. For our part we did not have any of those gifts bestowed upon us on that occasion, but we rejoiced greatly..."*[17]

For those in the early Church, the Sacrament was a sacred occasion, in which the worthy were privileged to partake, and the unworthy were put out of the room in which such things as these were observed:

> *I believe I was the first person, with a young man whose name I have forgotten, who was present when they took what was called the sacrament up at the Morley house. They were in the habit of turning every body out of the door when they partook of the bread and wine, putting blankets up at the windows, shutting off the sight from without. They started a regular pow-pow, and when they got well going, then they opened the door and let us all come in again.*[18]

And, of course, in the House of the Lord at Kirtland, Ohio, the Sacrament was a regular feature, while the faithful were fed temporally, God fed them spiritually at the same time:

> *...when we had fasted for 24 hours and partaken of the Lord's Supper, namely a piece of Bread as big as your double fist, and half a pint of wine in the Temple, I was there and saw the Holy Ghost descend upon the heads of those present like cloven tongues of fire.*[19]

Even the early missionaries of the Church used wine when conducting Sunday services in small branches over which they presided. Evan Melbourne Green relates an instance in 1833, where "we met in the

P.M. at Bro. W.'s house for the purpose of confirming those who were baptized on Sunday. Brother J administered the bread and wine to the little Church in this place. The Lord poured out His Spirit in a good degree."[20]

Wine was not just confined for secular use alone, but applied to other types of special events as well. Oliver Cowdery makes an entry in his "Sketchbook," of Wednesday, Janaury 20, 1836 as follows: "Copied blessings until evening, at which time I went, in company with my wife, to Elder John F. Boynton's wedding; a large company assembled, and after the services we were treated *WITH WINE* and cake very sumptuously."[21]

And, upon another occasion, the Prophet himself had to attend two wedding celebrations at the same time:

> *Returned home and spent the afternoon. Towards evening President Cowdery returned from Columbus, the capital of the State. I could spend but little time with him, being under obligation to attend at Mrs. Wilcox's, to join Mr. John Webb and Mrs. Catherine Wilcox in matrimony; also Mr. Thomas Carrico and Miss Elizabeth Baker, at the same place; all of which I performed in the customary manner in the midst of a large assembly. We then partook of some refreshments, and our hearts were made glad with THE FRUIT OF THE VINE. This is according to the pattern set by our Savior Himself, and we feel disposed to patronize all the institutions of heaven.*[22]

It is interesting to see how Joseph Smith justified his actions in the consumption of wine upon this occasion. He merely called attention to the Savior's own indulgence of the same at the marriage feast in Cana, wherein he performed His first recorded miracle. And the Prophet said he was doing it "according to the pattern set by our Savior himself." If such were his reasons, who is there that can legitimately criticize his imbibement at this time?

Still, later on, in June of 1836, he recorded:

> *My father and Uncle John Smith started on a mission to visit the branches of the Church in the Eastern States, to set them in order, and confer on the brethren their patriarchal blessings. I took my mother and Aunt Clarissa (my Uncle John's wife), in a carriage, and accompanied them to Painsville, where we procured A BOTTLE OF WINE, broke bread, ate and drank, and parted AFTER THE ANCIENT ORDER, with the blessings of*

God.[23]

It was the custom in Bible times for a man to hospitably entertain his guests by providing them with bread and wine. Such a thing occurred in the Book of Judges (19:17-21), which only goes to prove that Joseph Smith was following an ancient custom and order of things, which the Lord approved of wholeheartedly.

However, the frequent use of wine seems to have led some to an inclination for other types of alcoholic beverages too. These were generally consumed in quiet leisure, or taken as a form of "tawdy" when ill. Though the Prophet did not denounce these things in any strong terms, his counselor, Sidney Rigdon, did.

> *December 4, 1836, Sunday. I went up to the house of the Lord to worship. Elder Parrish preached in the forepart of the day. Several spoke in the latter part of the day. President Rigdon called a vote of the Church to discountenance the use entirely of all liquors from the Church in sickness and in health, except wine at the Sacraments and for external washing. The vote was carried unanimously. I spent the night with Elder Parrish.*[24]

Less than four months after this orthodox proposal by Sidney, we find the first substitution for wine mentioned in the annals of Church history: "At half-past five, bread and *WATER* were distributed liberally among the quorums, and it was truly a refreshing season to spirit and body."[25] Despite this new introduction, wine would still continue to be used in the Mormon sacraments until the turn of the century, when a new kind of "adaptation," would replace the "old distinctiveness" as first introduced by Joseph Smith.[26]

It was not until the summer of 1838 that the Prophet gave the Latter-day Saints a true pattern of how the Sacrament should be administered. This correct representation of the Lord's supper was revealed to them at Far West, Missouri sometime in June or July of that year.

> *The people came together in the morning without their breakfast, to the bowery on the Public Square where there was prepared a plenty of good bread and a barrel of WINE. The bread and wine was blessed, every person ate bread and DRANK WINE as they wanted ALL DAY, when they wanted. They sat and talked, and walked and conversed upon heavenly and spiritual things as they felt like. Walked out on the Prairie and returned to eat and drink.*

> *No one said, "Let's go and get a drink," but with solemnity they commemorated the death and sufferings of Jesus. A part of the day Joseph was preaching in the large room on the North side of the square, while George A. Smith preached on the South side, from a wagon; NO ONE WAS INTOXICATED during the day.*[27]

From this interesting narrative we learn one fact: *THE SAINTS WERE ABLE TO PARTAKE OF THE WINE ALL DAY LONG WITHOUT ANY OUTWARD SIGNS OF INEBRIATING EFFECT*! This would mean only one thing then, that the wine made by them for these purposes was LOW IN ALCOHOLIC CONTENT, and similar to that of ancient vintage. In other words, if the Sacrament had been restored according to an old pattern, most certainly the kind of drink used then would be revealed, too. And, as Dean Farrar has already mentioned, the beverages of antiquity "were more like syrups; many of them not intoxicant." Thus, it would be safe to conclude that the Latter-day Saints made their wine after the same gentle manner, thus producing a product similar in tartness to our present day buttermilk. Such a dairy item is only cultured to a certain point, after which it is packaged and sold. It is not allowed to develop to the stage that, say, something like clabbered milk would get. The same principle holds true with the Mormon blend of grape juice. It was permitted fermentation, but only to a slight degree. For how else could so many people consume so much in just one day without any noticeable side effects of lasting duration? It could never be done unless the wine was only *PARTIALLY AGED*. This explains the Lord's permission for them to use such things in their services. Had they been anything but mild, *HE WOULD NEVER HAVE ALLOWED IT!*

The advantages of making their own wine were many. At least they knew what ingredients went into the processing thereof. The Lord knew what He was doing when He gave them the commandment to that effect some years earlier. However, that did not always solve the problem of deadly matter being put into their vintage, for the enemies of the Church were numerous in those days, and no place could be found safe enough from their evil designs. Yet, if such a foul act of wickedness were committed upon an unsuspecting group of Saints, the Lord would nevertheless sanctify the sacramental emblems to the extent that whatever harmful agent had been secretly put in them would pass without avail through the systems of the partakers.

> *St. Mark, Chapter 16, verses xvii and xviii, "And these signs shall follow them that believe; in my name they shall cast out devils; they shall speak with new tongues; they shall take up*

serpents; and if they DRINK ANY DEADLY THING, IT SHALL NOT HURT THEM; they shall lay hands on the sick, and they shall recover."

In the year 1840 and 1841, the Elders of the Church of Jesus Christ of Latter-day Saints visited the little town of Grafton, Lorian Co., Ohio, and there they raised up a small branch, consisting of sixteen members. In the summer of 1841 this branch of the Church held their meetings in a building that was used on week days as a carpenter's shop, and consequently was open most of the time, having no lock or key.

On Sunday, towards the latter part of the summer of 1841, the teacher fetched the sacrament as usual, bread and wine (the wine being his own make from elderberries). He left the bread and wine in a basket under one of the work benches while he went to dinner.

In the afternoon sixteen persons partook of the same. When he returned home he took the decanter containing the wine out of the basket, and unthinking held it up between him and the sun when he discovered quite a quantity of sediment in it. This astonished him very much, for when he put the wine into the decanter it was perfectly clear.

He said nothing about it to anyone, but the next day he took it to a chemist and had it analyzed. It was found to contain about an ounce of ARSENIC! And sixteen persons drank of that poisoned wine, the writer of this sketch among the rest, and not one realized any injury. Thus we saw and realized the fulfillment of the promise, "if you drink any deadly thing it shall not hurt you."

But the offending party thought the joke too good to keep. In about three months after, a very sickened young man in the town said the Mormons could not be killed for he had tried it. Said he, "I put an ounce of arsenic in their sacramental wine and they partook of it and it did them no harm." His name was Dhru Johnson. In about four months after this circumstance transpired he quarreled with a man in a ballroom and was stabbed and killed.[28]

The custom of using wine for sacramental purposes was also carried into foreign lands by the Elders of the Church. When brothers

Young, Kimball, Pratt, Smith, and Hedlock landed in Liverpool, England, on Monday, April 6, 1840, after a tedious passage of twenty-eight days they "then went to No. 8 Union Street, where they procured bread and wine in order to partake of the Sacrament."[29]

As we have already learned, different kinds of fruit were used for wine, among which was red currants from Newel Knight's orchard in Kirtland, and the above-mentioned elderberry. As the Saints became more settled in their new home at Nauvoo, they were able to grow a variety of things. One such item was Concord grapes. The Icarians, who came after the Mormons, successfully cultivated these luscious berries, and to this day some of their remarkable vineyards still continue to grow in the City of Joseph.

The soil was perfect and the conditions right for their growth, and those who grew such fruit prospered indeed. In the month of November, 1845, on the last day of that season, the Nauvoo Brass Band "met at the residence of Brother B. Young, and played a few tunes; after which some excellent cake and wine were served; the cake and wine were excellent, *THE WINE BEING MADE OF THE PURE GRAPE, OF NAUVOO MANUFACTURE.*" And, at another occasion, the following February, of 1846, "the band met in the upper room of the Temple, by request of Brother B. Young.... During the evening they handed round some of *OUR NAUVOO GRAPE WINE*, which was excellent."[30]

And "on the 30th of September, 1845, General Hardin with 400 troops, arrived in Nauvoo....

"The Temple, the Masonic Hall, the Nauvoo House, and the stables of the Mansion House were then searched by General Hardin and his troops, for the ostensible purpose of finding the dead bodies spoken of. They found in the Masonic Hall, not dead bodies, but—about *FORTY BARRELS OF WILD GRAPE WINE,* which they fondly lingered about and devoted considerable attention to."[31]

Apparently, the general and his men liked the taste of the Mormon wine, for they seem to have spent an unusual length of time around the barrels, as if to imply that what they partook of caressed their senses of taste wonderfully well as a fair, young damsel would. One Utah writer, in referring to this historical incident, casually added a tongue-in-cheek apostrophe after the narrative: "He is trampling out the vintage where the grapes of wrath are stored."[32] Needless to say, the military authority departed that place with a favorable impression of Mormon culture.

The frequent use of wine in their Sacraments caused many Latter-day Saints to partake of it upon other occasions as well. Elder Jesse C. Little, who had been sent to Washington, D.C. by President Young to seek for government aid, relates that "I called upon Col. Kane...After drinking a glass of superior wine together, we separated. I left my blessing with him..."[33] In this instance, it was considered a social custom of good grace, and more for the hospitality extended him by his kind host did Elder Little feel to drink this, than for the wine itself. And, in another case involving Joseph Smith, was wine consumed, only for very different reasons. Brigham Young once made the observation:

> *If a person is weary, worn out, CAST DOWN, fainting, or dying, brandy sling, A LITTLE WINE, or a cup of tea is GOOD TO REVIVE THEM. Do not throw these things away, and say they must never be used; THEY ARE GOOD TO BE USED WITH JUDGMENT, PRUDENCE, AND DISCRETION.*[34]

For this purpose then was a little "fruit of the vine" slipped into Carthage Jail, to gladden the hearts of those who were incarcerated there. Elder John Taylor relates the circumstances behind this particular time, in these graphic words:

> *Sometime after dinner we sent for some WINE. It has been reported by some that this was taken as a sacrament. It was no such thing; our spirits were generally dull and heavy, and it was sent for to REVIVE US. I think it was Captain Jones who went after it, but they would not suffer him to return. I believe WE ALL DRANK OF THE WINE, and gave some to one or two of the prison guards. We, all of us, felt unusually dull and languid, with a remarkable depression of spirits. In consonance with those feelings I sang a song, that had lately been introduced into Nauvoo, entitled, 'A Poor Wayfaring Man of Grief,' etc.*[35]

Now the question arises, "Did Joseph Smith break the Word of Wisdom on this occasion?" We know not the proof of the vintage, nor the alcoholic content of the substance in mention; all we know about it is that it was not for sacramental purposes. This question can, perhaps, best be answered from the scriptures themselves.

In the Ten Commandments which God gave ancient Israel was this injunction:

> *Remember the sabbath day to keep it holy.*

Six days shalt thou labor, and do all thy work; But the seventh day is the sabbath of the Lord thy God; in it thou shalt not do any work. [36]

Now, they who administered the law unto the people, the Scribes and the Pharisees, placed the strict interpretation of *ALL WORK* upon it. To them, any sort of effort or physical labor, no matter for what purpose it may have been, was to be considered as *WORK*, and therefore, in violation of the Sabbath Day. Thus did they criticize Jesus and his disciples in the following manner once:

At that time Jesus went on the Sabbath day through the corn; and his disciples were an hungered, and began to pluck the ears of corn and to eat.

But when the Pharisees saw them, they said unto him, Behold, thy disciples do that which IS NOT LAWFUL to do upon the Sabbath day.[37]

And Jesus answered them by referring to the account of David, wherein "he was an hungered, and they that were with him." And related how David "entered into the house of God, and did eat the shewbread, which was *NOT LAWFUL* for him to eat, neither for them that were with him; but only for the priests."[38]

From this classic statement of the Saviour's, we are given to understand that what God commands and man interprets are two different things. The Word of Wisdom is a sound piece of advice from God, adopted by the Church as commandment later on. What Latter-day Saints read into it may be very different from the understanding in which the Almighty revealed it. Generally, the "letter" of the law is man's own doing, while the "spirit" of the thing comes from God. In this sense, then, were Joseph Smith and his brethren justified in what they did. Or, as the Lord so aptly put it: "Let no one, therefore, set on my servant Joseph; for *I WILL JUSTIFY HIM*!"[39]

To show just how wine may "revive the spirits," as Brigham suggests it can, the following anecdote is provided for that purpose:

My mother was born March 20, 1859 at Ephraim, Utah...

As a little girl, Maria J. Averett was left to care for the family of smaller children, while her mother helped earn the livelihood. I remember hearing her relate the following incident:

One day while her mother was gone, the child discovered a keg of wine stowed away in a corner. Being curious, she decided to taste it. She had no way of knowing that the liquid sucked directly from the "bung" is much more potent than when poured first into a glass, so she just stooped down and drank some of the wine right out of the spout. In a short time she became VERY HAPPY and when her mother returned and learned what had happened, she was shocked at such behaviour, scolded the child soundly and promised, "Just wait 'till I tell your father." Maria waited in terrified anticipation of what might happen when her father learned of her disgraceful conduct. When he arrived, she was cold sober, but when he heard the story, he just laughed and said, "Was it good, daughter?" Never again did she have any desire to imbibe.[40]

Scarcely had the Saints settled in their new home than plans were already being laid, on a large scale basis, for future wineries:

Early in the year 1851, the Church conceived the idea of manufacturing wine and olive oil for Sacrament purposes, consequently they made a call for a company of 100 men to go to Southern California for the purpose of planting grape vines and olive trees, from which to manufacture the olive oil and wine. Father, Uncle David, with their families and Edwin left for Southern California March 15, 1851, and arrived at Siccimore Grove at the mouth of Cahoon Pass, June 11, 1851, and settled in San Bernardino the same year. They planted ten acres of grape vines east of the Santianna River what was called the old San Bernardino Catholic Mission, now called Smilly Heights. They then sold the vine yard to a man by the name of Aldrich and built a saw mill on the head waters of a stream that emptied into the Mohava River. They operated this mill until their departure for Utah again.[41]

However, after some further consideration of the matter, it was deemed in the best wisdom to confine such things in a more localized area, where they would be under better control of the people:

President Young had designated the country of Dixie as most congenial for the raising of grapes and for experimental projects in cotton. Knowing of John Conrad Naegle's skill in wine distillery, in which Konrad Kleinman had often aided him, they were appointed to look after that industry and thus the finest grapes grown in the state flourished in Dixie, from which

> *vast quantities of wine and fine distilled brandies were made. The latter to supply the drug stores in the cities with alcohol for the preservation of medicines. The wine was used EXTENSIVELY in the Sacrament services, as in olden times, being stored in immense vats or caks in the basement of the Naegle home until it could be freighted by team to Salt Lake City.*[42]

Brigham Young felt as his predecessor had done, that wine was good for the sacred purpose of the sacrament, provided "it be made by our own hands."[43] However, he was aware of the fact that some of the people took a regular liking to this holy emblem, and would consume more than what duty or wisdom required. So, he felt to admonish some of them in St. George on May 1, 1869: "I have no doubt were we to offer the Wine in sacrament that some would swallow a Pint if the tumbler would (hold) that much before they could bite it off. However, I (can) remedy that. I will have tumblers made that will just hold a swallow and no more."[44]

Wine was used for many years in the Sacrament at the Tabernacle on Temple Square. An interesting story is connected with the wine goblets used by the members then:

> *James H. Barlow was one of the first jewelers in Salt Lake City, and his work was of the highest order. He made the most intricate designs in long earrings, so popular in those days, bracelets, rings, brooches, etc. Many expensive and much prized heirlooms in Utah's First Families are his handiwork.*
>
> *Many of the Saints who had come to Utah had been wealthy. Travelling as they did by ox teams or handcarts, they could not bring much of their earthly possessions. Material things such as fine linens, china, books, and furniture had to be left behind. Their jewels they could carry along, and they did. A call was made by the leaders of the Church for all the silver ornaments anyone would like to give. In the days when Moses was busy on Mount Sinai, a call went forth for all the jewels both silver and gold. With that, was made an idol of a calf to be worshipped. These jewels were put to a more acceptable use. They were made by James K. Barlow into a Sacrament Service to be used in the Tabernacle. These consisted of shallow baskets for the bread and cups for the wine. These cups were about six inches high and had handles on opposite sides to facilitate the passing frcm one person to the next. These were used for many years, until a more sanitary method was discovered and each participant had an individual cup.*

> *After the large silver cups were discarded they were distributed among the Barlow children. Kate had one which she proudly displays as the workmanship of her Father. He had his office and shop in the home and she used to like to slip in and watch him at work with the bright shining gold and silver and the precious stones he used in making up his expensive jewelry.*[45]

Often when the Saints would handle these emblems, their minds and thoughts would be elsewhere. As such, Heber C. Kimball offered several recommendations to the people, which would prove helpful to them if they followed it and adopted such wise counsel into their lives. For then the observance would take on a whole new meaning entirely and generate an appreciation within the soul for sacred things now considered rather common.

> *We are now partaking of the sacrament of the Lord's Supper; when we partake of the bread, let us pray the Father that strength may be given to our bodies that they may not wither, but be strengthened to reach a good old age; when we partake of the wine which is emblematic of his blood, let us ask the Father that our blood may never be spilled unless it is necessary for the advancement of his Kingdom and the glory of God.*[46]

When such advice was not followed, sickness would be the result, or a spiritual lethargy, which would leave the unhappy victim in a stupor of thought as to the things of God. So said an apostle of the Lord in 1890, when he "showed the importance of partaking of the Sacrament of the Lord's Supper worthily." This same apostle said that "he would as soon take a cup of poison as to take it unworthily." further showed that many were sick among the people and some slept on that account."[47]

A meal was not considered complete without some flavorful wine to liven the occasion a bit:

> *We had a brave long grace before meat. I noticed that before uttering it President Young's eye had wandered over the table, to see every corner lifted, even the glass top of the butter-dish. The stoppers were taken from the decanters of HOMEMADE WINE.*[48]

And even the first great prophet of this last dispensation was well remembered in rousing toasts:

Thursday, December 23, 1880. Anniversary of the birth of Joseph Smith... In the afternoon was a public meeting at the tabernacle in commemoration of the birth of the great and mighty Seer, Joseph Smith.

...In the evening, I took my wife and daughter Nelly to the evening entertainment at St. George hall... The hall was filled with the picked faithful saints of St. George. Speeches were made by some good speakers upon the rise of the Church...

After speeches, music by band and organ, songs and reading poems, cakes and apples were freely passed. After that WINE was passed until all had drunk all they desired and yet NO ONE SHOWED SIGNS OF INTOXICATION; that is the part most surprising to me. I have seen food passed and speeches, etc., made but I never before saw 200 or more people with free access to STRONG DRINK and no one to be seen intoxicated.[49]

Here we have the first indication as to the potency of this Utah-made beverage. Apparently the Saints let their territorial wine age a little more than what they had done in Nauvoo or other places previous to this. However, it is to their lasting credit that self-restraint was practiced and prudence used when partaking of such "strong drink." After all, the man whom they were honoring had practiced temperance in his lifetime, and certainly the finest tribute which could be paid to him would be for his disciples to imitate these same virtues and apply them into their own lives as well. Thus, among the more faithful part of the people, a temperate Prophet begat a temperate people.

As more of the younger generation born in Utah grew up, certain things within the Mormon theology were replaced with other things. The Manifesto ended plural marriage, for example, thus allowing for less Federal restriction unjustly imposed upon the people by the United States government, and gave way to new freedoms to be enjoyed by the Latter-day Saints. What had been a territory for so many years now became a full-fledged state and was admitted into the Union January 4, 1896. And, in some areas of Utah, water began to take the place of wine as a "new image" of a more "positive" approach to Mormonism slowly took shape.

However, despite these gradual changes, wine was still used for religious purposes among the leadership of the Church.

When the brethren returned, we clothed in our robes and

F.D. Richards prayed and we knelt and President Snow at the altar, we then dressed in our usual clothing and prepared to eat the Lord's Supper in the same manner in which the Prophet Joseph said it was eaten by the Savior and His disciples at Jerusalem, and as Joseph and the brethren did occasionally at Nauvoo, we had several loaves of bread and BOTTLES OF WINE. The former was broken—and we ate and drank till we were fully satisfied. I took a very small quantity of wine.[50]

The passing of fermented grape beverage in the Mormon religion came about in a quiet, dignified manner. Rather than an edict being issued decrying the use of this anymore, it was allowed to be "phased" from the program of things in a very natural sort of way. Or, as one commentator so effectively put it:

Until 1900 there were numerous references to the use of wine in the Sacrament but after the turn of the century the communion goblet and the wine glass were put reverently aside to appear no more in the Mormon worship service.[51]

Now that we have carefully examined the secular use of wine in Mormon theology, let us take a moment and look at another aspect in which this found good service—namely, in the medicinal end of things for purposes of health and well-being.

For several thousand years, wine has formed a base for certain medicines to be made in. The noted physician Galen "was a strong believer in the therapeutic value of wine and recommended that no wines be drunk unless at least seven years of age. It is said that wines which had been aged for a century were not uncommon at the tables of wealthy Romans of this time."[52] Whether such drinks of dynamite proof remedied a malady or not is uncertain. However, one thing of which we can be sure: the patient didn't care if he was cured or not after swallowing a generous dose of the doctor's prescription. In other words, "he was feeling no pain."

The Apostle Paul urged Timothy to use a little wine for internal disorders: "Drink no longer water, but *USE A LITTLE WINE* for thy stomach's sake and thine often infirmities."[53]

An American nutrition expert of the 1930s shared Paul's belief by this medical observation:

...one of the best dietaries possible is that typified by the French table d'hote dinner; many an American who thought he

had chronic digestive troubles has been surprised to find them disappear when he spent two or three weeks on first rate French food, including the dry (not sweet) vin ordinaire in a country where wine is wine and not a factory processed soft drink plus added alcohol...

The extensive use of wines at every meal, as is practiced in many parts of Europe, is not a bad habit, as it is regarded by...many...moral factors in our American civilization; wine drinking was one of those vital adjustments made by man to an imperfect food and water supply. A diet high in spaghetti, macaroni, and other pastas and devoid of the native wine of Italy or France would not be merely indigestible but would be dangerous to health and mental activity.[54]

In the Middle Ages wine found its way into the apothecary with such remedies as crushed strawberry leaves taken with distilled water or wine for "passion of the heart," and "reviving the spirits," a process that the herbalists declared "maketh the hert merrie."[55]

Early Mormon botanic specialists such as Dr. William Decator Kartchner relied quite extensively upon spiritous liquors and wine as a proper solution to help the medicine go down a bit easier:

On the 6th day of June, 1879, I took sick with a pain in the bowels and dropsy developed. On June 28, I attended conference and got worse. Kept to my bed for sometime. On September 4, I was able to sit up a little. My neighbors and acquaintances' proposed several remedies and every one applied seemed to help me, 'among which was bitter aloes in whiskey for a purgative and the wild milkweed root in whiskey—large tablespoonful every six hours for a few days, then every morning until I was well; also grapevine bark ashes, a teaspoonful IN A LITTLE WINE every morning. In five days seven gallons of water ran through me through the natural channel. Up until January, 1880, I continued to take the milkweed root, which is the best of all the remedies.[56]

In fact, towards the closing moments of his mortal life, President John Taylor resorted to a little fermented drink in order to ease the pain and make things a bit more pleasant for him all around:

Tuesday, July 5, 1887—...President Taylor arose early this morning. He said he was some better and felt quite hopeful.

He, however, didn't eat anything. Sister Pricilla Jennings sent a letter accompanied by two bottles of homemade wine to the President. He tasted the wine and seemed to enjoy it.[57]

And in the Smith family itself wine became a procurative factor in the healing of one Lovisa Mack Tuttle, sister to Lucy Mack Smith, the Prophet's mother. Solomon Mack, Joseph Smith's grandfather on his mother's side of the family, related the strange circumstances surrounding her sudden recovery, in his little known *Narrative*:

For three days she (ate) only the yoke of one egg; she was an anatomy to appearance. Her friends were often weeping around her bed, expecting every moment to be her last. The day before her recovery, the doctor said it was as much impossible to raise her, as it would from the dead.

The night following she dreamed a dream; it was that a sort of wine would cure her. It was immediately brought to her, and she drank it. The next morning she awoke and called to her husband to get up and make a fire. He arose immediately, but thought she was out of her head. But soon he found to the contrary. Quickly she arose up on end in the bed, said the Lord has helped both body and soul, and dressed herself. She then asked for the Psalm Book and turned to the 30th Psalm, second part (readers look for yourselves), and again she mentioned the 116th, first part.[58]

Even in our present age "wine is considerably used in pharmacy as a menstruum, and, with a qualifying phrase or word indicating the medicinal substance dissolved, the word (cf. vinum) appears in the names of many solutions; as, *wine* of opium; orange *wine*, etc."[59]

Today the leaders of the Mormon Church frown upon the use of wine, in any form, by its members. It is no longer used in their sacraments, and is strictly forbidden as a consumptive agent. Housewives are encouraged to abstain from the use of wine in any culinary dishes, which may call for such a thing in the ingredients. A recent Church editorial stressed the point in this fashion:

Almost daily in the women's departments of newspapers recipes are provided for various food items. Invariably some recipes call for the use of wine... What should be the attitude of the Latter-day Saint housewife regarding the use of such recipes? ...Are we not bright enough to recognize that putting

> *liquor into food is just another means devised by the distillers to increase their sales? Will we be duped by such a device? And anyway, should Latter-day Saints even have liquor in the home UNDER ANY GUISE?*[60]

Considering that today's wine has many chemical additives, and is processed with a higher marginal allowance of alcohol in it than what God would approve of, the present views of modern day prophets should be sustained and obeyed. And, in accordance with God's original commandment to Joseph Smith to not use any wine "save it be that of your own make" and Brigham Young's sage advice that "such things (as homemade wine) ought not to be done away with, but retained as medicine," together with the Apostle Paul's admonition, "Use a little wine for thy stomach's sake," it would be well for Latter-day Saints to wait upon the Lord in this matter, until He again reveals His will unto them concerning the use of pure, homemade vintage and its rightful place among our people.

NOTES

1. *JD* 4:78.

2. *Ibid.*

3. Lafayette C. Lee, *op., cit.* (Previous chapter notes).

4. Webster's, *op. cit.*, p. 2933 (Previous chapter notes).

5. *JD* 4:78.

6. *JD* 19:92.

7. William Smith, *A Dictionary of the Bible*; Philadelphia, 1948; p. 747.

8. *D&C* 89:7.

9. Leviticus 10:8—10.

10. Judges 13:4.

11. *DHC* 1:78.

12. *D&C* 27:2.

13. *Ibid.*, 3.

14. McGavin, list. D&C, *op., cit.*, pp 84-85 (Previous chapter notes).

15. *Woman's Exponent* 7:71, 83 (October 1, 1878, #9; November 1, 1878, #7).

16. *DHC* 1:334—335.

17. Ebenezer Robinson, "Items of Personal History of the Editor," *The Return*, I (June 1889), Davis City, Iowa; pp. 88-91.

18. Braden, Clark and Kelly, E.L.; *Public Discussion of the Issues Between the Reorganized Church of Jesus Christ of Latter-day Saints and the Church of Christ, Disciples, Held in Kirtland, Ohio*: St. Louis, Missouri, 1884; pp. 383—384.

    A Church historian mentions that in 1831 at a log dwelling owned by Isaac Morley "even the door was muffled with cloths to prevent a noise" while Joseph and the Elders prayed for a sick woman who was immediately healed. (Andrew Jenson, *The Historical Record;* Salt Lake, 1886; p. 136).

19. Charles L. Walker Diary, p. 665; Harold B. Lee Library, BYU, Provo.

20. Evan M. Greene's Journal (January 15, 1833 - April 1 1835), Thursday 19th entry. Church Historian's Office, Salt Lake City.

21. BYU Studies, Summer 1972, p. 417.

22. *DHC* 11:369.

23. *Ibid.*, pp. 446—447.

24. BYU Studies, Summer, 1972; p. 373.

25. *DHC* 11:480.

26. Nels Anderson, *Desert Saints*; Chicago, 1942; pp. 443, 445.

27. *History of the Life of Oliver B. Huntington*, by Oliver B. Huntington; pp. 31-32. Privately published, no date, no place of publication.

28. *Woman's Exponent* 12:29, as submitted by Joanna C. Teeples, Holdin, Utah, June 15, 1883.

29. *DHC* 4:104.

30. *The Contributor* 1:196-197.

31 Jenson, *op., cit.*, p 822

32. LaMar Petersen, *Hearts Made Glad*; Salt Lake, 1975; p. 198.

33. Journal History, July 6, 1846, p. 5. Church Library, Salt Lake City.

34. *JD* 12:403 (28).

35. *DHC* 7:101.

36. Exodus 20:8-10 (Inspired Version).

37. Matthew 12:1-2.

38. *Ibid.*, 3—4.

9. *D&C* 132:59.

40. Maria J.A. Shumway, Robert Clayton Collection, *op., cit.*, fd. #152, bx. 3.

41. Material in possession of the author.

42. Anna Benz Kleinman, Robert Clayton, *op., cit.*, fd. #84, bx. 1.

43. *JD* 19:92.

44. Robert Glass Cleland and Juanita Brooks, *A Mormon Chronicle: The Diaries of John D. Lee;* San Marino, California: The Huntington Library; 1955; Volume II, pp. 116-117.

45. "History of Mesa—Catherine Barlow Burton," Roberta Clayton Collection, *op., cit.*, fd. #14, bx.1.

46. *JD* 10:102—103.

47. Charles L. Walker, *op., cit.*, p. 924.

48. Sarah Wood Kane, *Twelve Mormon Homes Visited In Succession on a Journey Through Utah to Arizona;* Philadelphia, 1874.

49. Oliver B. Huntington, *op., cit.*, p. 4.

50. Abraham H. Cannon Journals, p. 123; Harold B. Lee Library, BYU, Provo, Utah.

51. Peterson, *op., cit.*, p. 114.

52. Charles H. La Wall, *The Curious Lore of Drugs and Medicines* (Four Thousand Years of Pharmacy); New York, 1927; p. 66.

53. I Timothy 5:25.

54. F. J. Schlink, *Eat Drink, and Be Wary*; New York,1935; pp,. 283, 286.

55. *Natural History* magazine, December 1959, p. 590.

56. DUP Lesson for October 1957, "And They Were Healed," p. 108; by Kate B. Carter.

57. *Diary of L. John Nutall*, p. 98. Harold B. Lee Library, BYU, Provo, Utah.

58. Solomon Mack, *A Narrative of the Life of Solomon Mack*; Windsor, Vermont, 1811 (?).

59. *Webster's, op., cit.*, p. 2933.

60. *Church News*, March 17, 1973, p. 16.

See "Joseph Smith and His Progenitors" by Lucy Mack Smith, pp. 12-15, for a more detailed account of Lovisa Tuttle's sickness and subsequent return to full and proper health. It will be noted that mention of the dream concerning the wine has been omitted from Mother Smith's work; but she does say on the top of page 14, that Lovisa requested "her husband to bring her some wine, saying, if he would do so she would do quite well for the present." Also missing is the scripture she read when upon her feet once again. However, Mother Smith's account is more detailed than her father's was, for she relates the heavenly vision which Lovisa had while in the Spirit World, and also of seeing the Savior and the instructions He gave her.

For a comparative study of the two accounts, consult Richard L. Anderson's, "Joseph Smith's New England Heritage," pp. 76-77.

CHAPTER SIX

LIVING LIKE CRUSOE

(Tropical Fruit, Nuts, and Berries as Mormon Food)

On a faraway island by the sea,

Robinson Crusoe lived quite free;

He ate of the bounties that Nature provides,

Mangoes and oranges and banana-skin hides.

Now mangoes make sense, and citrus does too,

But when asked on the third, replied Mister Crusoe,

"Oh, the mangoes I like and the citrus I love,

But those banana-skin hides help to give them a shove."[1]

Very little is said about fruits, nuts, and berries in the Mormon diet. Material is scarce and hard to find when searching the records for mention of these things among the pioneers. However, the efforts of labor were rewarded in a slight "find" of an early missionary's journal, in which is faithfully recounted an accurate record of what he and his companion ate while assigned to the Society Islands, Tahiti, and Bora-Bora from 1899 until 1902. Elder C. J. Hansen of Collinston, Utah, provides an interesting glimpse into the lives of two Mormon preachers as they find that remote paradise is not all it is cracked up to be. That, in fact, the natives could be rather lazy, thus disproving the theory about having a savage house-boy named Friday to do all the work for you.

The following excerpts taken from his diaries contain an assorted list of practically all the food he ate while residing there. Everything from coconuts to pineapples, roast suckling pig to wormy chicken soup, is mentioned below. After the reader has gone through this man's narrative, he will better appreciate the natural fruits which our missionary friend ate while there. Because considering everything *ELSE* which he consumed in the meantime, the other seems to have been his lifesaver in cleansing his system from all the impurities of the unnatural foods he took within his body.

> *March 30, 1899—Landed at Papatee. Went to Missionary Headquarters. Slept on the floor with nothing but a quilt under me. I got but very little sleep...I had the blues plenty.*
>
> *March 31, 1899—Woke up in a strange land. Thirteen of us sat down to breakfast. We had nothing but bread and water for breakfast. Went down to the ship and got a piece of mutton and a potato. Felt blue and hungry. Started to live on native fruits and sweet potatoes. Started to cheer up toward night. Three years looks like an age. Almost feel like going back home and letting Canackes go to the devil.*
>
> *April 14, 1899—Papatee Tahiti—My birthday—21 years old... Bought a franc's worth of candy to celebrate the event. We also had some coconuts and pineapples...*
>
> *May 1, 1899—Papatee —I stopped at a house and bought some coconuts to drink. The coconut water is delicious. When we got back to headquarters we were very tired. Ate a can of beef and some bread for supper...*
>
> *Sunday, May 7, 1899—Fast day; went to 3 meetings; felt somewhat blue... Took a walk with Brother Taylor & Doudle. Visited the ship 'Tropic Bird'; had a drink of claret wine with the ship's cook.*
>
> *May 9, 1899—Papatee Tahiti—My turn to cook; gave the brethren some rice for breakfast; got some tomatoes and onions for dinner with some sweet potatoes and coconut milk. It makes a capital soup!*
>
> *June 17, 1899—Visited Mr. Clausen and had all the bananas and oranges that I could eat.*
>
> *July 4, 1899—Borabora—The glorious fourth. No cannon woke us from our slumbers. We were invited to dinner by Messrs. Clausen and Elliott. We first held our usual morning prayers and then retired to an orange grove and partook of the luscious fruit to about a dozen a piece. We were then ready for breakfast. The meal consisted of chicken soup, hard tack, roasted pig, green corn, coconut water and milk, bread fruit,*

swine, chicken, taro and pumpkin... We enjoyed the meal as only Mormon missionaries can!

July 14, 1899—Borabora—Brother Hatch, McG. and I were invited to breakfast by the Governor. We were served in French style. The main thing for breakfast was beef, which was served different ways. All the white men and Governors of districts were in attendance. We also had bread, the first I had tasted for a month.

July 17, 1899—Borabora—Visited Clausen's on our return and he gave us a bunch of bananas...

July 20, 1899—Borabora—I took a walk to town after some bread, the first that had been for sale since I struck the town. We hailed it with delight...

July 26, 1899—Borabora—Cook day! Was busy all day. I first went up to Clausen's and got some oranges and onions. Went to town and bought a bottle of coal oil. I then killed a chicken and made a fine soup, but owing to it being fast day, I was weary before dinner was finally served...

August 4, 1899—Borabora—My cook day. I made a chicken soup...

August 7, 1899—Borabora—My cook day. I had a terrible time cooking some bread fruit on the fire. I was nearly smoked out.

August 16, 1899—Fast day, my cook day. Went to town and got some eggs and bread.

September 11, 1899—Borabora—My cook day. Took a walk up to the store and bought a can of beef, some rice, and eggs. On the way home, the rice sprung a leak. I had quite a time tying it up again.

September 15, 1899—The native gave us plenty of nice coconuts to drink and oranges.

September 29., 1899—My cook day. Stayed home and tended to my work. We nearly starved for supper; all we had was eggs in yams.

October 7, 1899—Went up town; bought some coal oil,

honey, and bread... Carried a large bunch of bananas from Clausen's that he gave me.

Monday, October 23, 1899—I went up to the store and purchased some beef, honey and bread for breakfast.

November 24, 1899—My cook day; went up town and bought some condinsed milk, bread and a can of egg plums.

December 2, 1899—My cook day; took a walk up town ard bought some bread. Mr. Ellicot gave us a pumpkin pie, which we highly appreciate.

Sunday, December 3, 1899—Held two meetings which were poorly attended and poorly appreciated; the natives all took a nap.

Monday, December 4, 1899—I took a walk up to Clatzsen's in afternoon and got a basket of mangoes.

Tuesday, December 5, 1899—Took a walk up to Clausen's and got some more mangoes. Had the blues; felt nervous all day...

January 1, 1900—Borabora—Brother E. T. Hatch and I were invited out to a native feast. The feast was spread on tables in a long house built for that purpose. We had chicken soup, bread, watermelon, and coffee...

We were next invited out to supper by Mr. Ellicot and, of course, we accepted without hesitating as us Mormons (Mendicants) always do. We had cabbage, soup, suckling pig with dressing, duck, tarrow, plum pudding, bread, claret wine, and coffee...

Tuesday, January 9, 1900—Borabora—It was our regular fast day, but we failed to observe it. We went fishing instead...and had a good old time. When the fish were divided, we got three big ones. Mrs. Ellicot gave us four more... We got home about four o'clock and had one of our fish broiled. They are out of sight that way, in short order...

January 13, 1900, Saturday—We went around to Anuai and back. We had nothing to eat, but mangoes until four o'clock, when we stopped with a native and got a fill up on fish and bread fruit...

Tuesday, January 23, 1900—We studied language in the forenoon and went to a native marriage in the afternoon...The marrying over, we went to the feast. We had fine soup, duck, chicken, pork, pie, bread, melon, coffee, poi. (They had about ten pigs in all). We enjoyed the meal immensely. After that we went, to the house of the groom, but we could not eat anymore seeing as how we were stuffed like the pigs they served. The relatives of both, give a feast and try to outdo each other by a lavish display of food...

April 18, 1900—Our regular fast day, but owing to not partaking of a spirit of fasting, without going against our feelings, we decided it best not to be hypocrites and fast as they do. So we took it upon ourselves to do away with that part of our work, without consulting higher authority in the matter.

May 23, 1900—I sailed for Maupiti...I took a can of sea biscuits with me. Also several cans of milk and beef...

May 25—26, 1900—Studied language; wrote out a sermon on repentance... I fasted the 26th for strength to hold a meeting and the language.

May 27, 1900—When I woke up I found I had caught a good cold in the head. My nose and mouth began to run water in streams, so I cancelled my meetings; went on the back porch and read a wild and wooly novel clear through.

May 28, 1900—I was doctoring my cold. I was kept awake hacking and coughing.

May 29, 1900—I was choked up till I had to breathe through my mouth. I get up to see what time it was and saw it was three o'clock. I went back to bed and slept till seven. When I got up and drank some hot ginger tea...I felt better. I also gave an old lady who was suffering with a terrible cancer, a cup of tea. I suppose she felt better right away, or at least it must have warmed her up... "Where the Lord has a house of prayer, the Devil will have a chapel there."

Sunday, June 17, 1900—They treated us very well...bringing me plenty of good food, poi, pork, etc.

Monday, June 18, 1900—I was also invited out to supper by Mr. Willie Ship, a friendly half-caste, and, of course, accepted as such invitations don't come often...We had a lavish display of food; we had pork, chicken, fish, liver, yams, bread fruit, and tea. It was fixed up to a queen's taste. The only trouble I had was to keep from eating too much, for when the natives fix up a feast, it is a feast indeed.

Maupiti, June 20, 1900—The natives gave me all the oranges, bananas and mangoes I could eat...

June 28, 1900—Went to Clausen's and had tea with him...

July 4, 1900—We were invited up to Clausen's to dinner together with the French Gendarme, Mr. Tropse, Mr. John Ellicot, Will Ellicot, Mr. Antone Ellicot. We sang the star-spangled banner; Brother Wright and I, also America, and the Soldier's Farewell. We drank the French absence, unfurled the stars and stripes and the French flag... Our dinner was grand—the best I have yet had in the South Seas. We had pork steak, roast pork, pork stew, chicken curry, chicken soup, omelet, fish, salad, cake, wine, cigarettes, and eggnog. We got (paia maitai roa) full!

July 5, 1900—Eating...dinner. It consisted of green plantaines, roasted in a fire. Green plaintaines are a very dry food; awful hard to swallow; potatoes would be way ahead of them for taste and strength...how one can work on such food beats me.

August 6, 1900—My cook day. We had yam stew, and eggs.

August 8, 1900—We were invited to Mr. Clausen's for dinner. We had an excellent dinner. We had fried turtle, chicken, young roast pig, yam coconuts, bananas, etc...

August 21, 1900, Tuesday—I made three visits to the sick. One was a case of paralysis—an old lady about 50. I gave her some ginger tea... The other was an infant suffering with a cramp in the stomach. I gave it some peppermint tea.

August 24, 1900—We bought a pig that weighed 90 pounds for $3.40...

August 27, 1900—I went to visit a sick man who had the lockjaw. I had quite a time getting some medicine for him. I gave him a dose of laudanum and poured hot oil into a sore on his foot, which caused the trouble. I afterwards put a poultice on the sore, which the natives removed as soon as I left because it pained him.

August 28, 1900—I called again upon the man, and had his foot lanced and probed for the coral rock which was supposed to be in his foot, but without success. I put on another poultice, which the natives again removed. I wanted to give him another dose of laudanum, but he would not consent. He was suffering terribly. He would first be drawn frontwards and then backwards. I could do nothing for him then, so took my medicine and left. That night, at two o'clock, he died.

October 18, 1900—I cooked a chicken for soup. I mixed some compressed soup of vegetables in it. The preparation was full of worms, which I had failed to notice. It was too much for Brother Earl; he did not want any soup, but I simply removed the worms and enjoyed it. I go by the taste, not by the looks!

Tuesday, October 23, 1900—I went up on the hill and got a nice basket of oranges. We afterwards bought a dozen pineapples and as we have plenty of bananas, we have high living at the white house.

November 1-5, 1900—I made several calls on the sick. I have run out of quinine and pain killer, my main medicines. I give them for everything from heart failure down to abortion.

January 15, 1901—Borabora—I made seven calls on the sick, but was unable to do anything for any of them. Most of them were children suffering with worms, supposed to be caused by eating mangoes. I am suffering with pin worms myself, but there is no medicine at hand. I have sent to Tahiti however, for some medicine with one of the traders.

February 14, 20, 1901—I got all ready to go to Railia and then backed out. I had to stand treat on that, to a can of pears and corn.

Ravahere, September 23, 1901—October 5, 1901—Natives treated or fed us very poorly. Anticipated better food after October 1, when the pearl diving commenced. Our hopes were realized as the natives started to bake bread, instead of the old "dough Gods" or boiled dumplings.

January 1, 1902—We had a big feast of pork and poi, which made us very sick. We both woke up during the night and began vomiting, and cussing the South Seas good. We pulled through all right; but do not hope to be invited to the New Year's in future, in any such a manner.[2]

In his last entry, Elder Hansen makes mention of an island dish romantically styled as 'poi.' But after one sampling of this pleasant-sounding food, the honeymoon is immediately over, and the stomach is ready to divorce it from the system entirely. Elder George Q. Cannon, who himself went on a mission to Hawaii in the summer of 1850, was well acquainted with the substance, and describes it fondly (?) in these appropriate words:

Before leaving Lahaina, I had tasted a teaspoonful of "poi"; but the smell of it and the calabash in which it was contained was so much like that of a book-binder's old, sour, paste-pot that when I put it to my mouth I gagged at it, and would have vomited had I swallowed it. But in travelling among the people I soon learned that if I did not eat 'poi' I would put them to great inconvenience; for they would have to cook separate food for me every meal. This would make me burdensome to them, and might interfere with my success. I, therefore, determined to learn to live on their food, and, that I might do so, I asked the Lord to make it sweet to me. My prayer was heard and answered; the next time I tasted it, I ate a bowlful, and I positively liked it. It was my food, whenever I could get it from that time as long as I remained on the islands.

It may sound strange, yet it is true, that I have sat down to a table on which bread was placed, and though I had not tasted the latter for months, I took the poi in preference to the bread; it was sweeter to me than any food I had ever eaten.[3]

Now, the South Sea Islanders had their own special way of eating this food. Brother Cannon describes the *petite* fashion in which they did so:

As soon as the blessing was asked, every one dipped his or her forefingers into the 'poi,' and lifting as much as the fingers would hold, they passed them into their mouths, throwing their heads back as they did so, to get a good mouthful.... The sucking of the fingers, the gusto with which they eat, and the incessant conversation mingled with laughter which they keep up, would lead a bystander to conclude that they enjoy this food. And they do...

We Elders who ate with them were also seated on mats and ate the same kind of food that they did, only in place of using our fingers we either used spoons or small paddles which we whittled out of wood, to convey the food to our mouths, thinking it would be better to set them an example in this respect.[4]

Another Mormon Elder who had similar experiences with this native dish was B. Morris Young, son of President Lorenzo Snow. He describes the celebration which he attended and the good things they ate, in this manner:

Now to the "big feast"—the old meeting house is not taken by surprise, but is trimmed and tastefully fitted for the doubly interesting occasion. On each side of the house tablecloths are spread on the floor, with plenty of ferns scattered around for the people to sit on; and on the tablecloths are spread poi in callow baskets, beef, pork, chicken, watermelons and bananas, on plates, but no plates, no knives and forks, and no spoons to eat with. We all ate as the Hawaiians do, with our fingers.[5]

For those who may not know what poi is, George Q. Cannon furnishes us with an accurate description of the same and how it is prepared:

This is made out of a root which they call kalo. "Kalo" patches are so made that they can be flooded with water; and the ground is never allowed to be uncovered. In planting this root they do not use seed. When a native gathers the "kalo," he carries it to his home, where he cuts off the tops. These are carefully saved, tied up in a bundle, and carried back to the patch. These tops he sticks in the mud at the proper distances apart, and at the end of about eleven months he has another crop of "kalo." This is the process of gathering and planting.

The "kalo" bears some resemblance in its leaves and taste to the wild Indian turnips, but its root is much larger; not quite the shape of a tame turnip, but as large as a moderate sized one. There is a variety called the "dry land kalo." It is not so extensively cultivated as the other kind, and is not considered so good eating.

Near every home there is a circular hole. When "kalo" is

cooked, a fire is built in this, and a quantity of small volcanic rocks are piled on top of it. As the fire burns out these sink to the bottom, and they are spread over the bottom and around the sides of the pit. The "kalo" roots are then laid in, mats are spread over them, then soil, until they are completely covered, excepting a small hole at the top, into which water is poured. That hole is then stopped, and the cooking commences.

"But how do they cook?" you may ask.

When the water is poured in, the rocks, being hot, speedily convert it into steam, and, as it cannot escape, it cooks the roots.

When the "kalo" has been in long enough to cook, it is uncovered; the skin is washed off, and it is pounded with a stone pestle, on a large flat slab of wood until it is like a mass of dough. Then it is put into a calabash, or gourd, and by the next day fermentation has commenced; or, as we would say if it were bread, it has "raised." Water is then added to it, and it is mixed until it is a little thinner than we usually make mush. There is a little sour taste about it the first day. But it is never eaten at that time by the natives, unless they have no other food. They like it best when it is quite sour. This is what they call "poi," and there is no other food that they think can equal it.[6]

Not all Latter-day Saints sent to the islands as missionaries were fortunate enough in finding a variety of things to eat. Some had to rough it a little, including delicate females:

After four days sail, landed at Kawhow, Hawaii, in the fall of 1851. Sister Elvira S. Barney lived for six months among the natives on their island food, mostly of taro and sweet-potatoes made into a batter and soured, short rations at that, yet attained the weight of one hundred and fifty pounds.[7]

The old adage that "Crusoe never had it so good" is more myth than reality. Sometimes the euphoric pleasures of constant feasting in Paradise would vanish into thin air when severe conditions of absolute starvation became quite evident:

Tropical islands usually abound in food throughout the year, but Elder Wood often found this to be more fancy than fact. For various reasons and at different times, he found himself without sufficient food, and often became painfully aware of it.

As water travel was so important in his work, he once spent all his money to buy a small boat and then records that he "had nothing to eat but crackers and not enough of that." Lack of food also resulted from the devastating native war, and again crackers became the main item of the diet. Some shark meat was graciously given to the Elders. One of them said he did not like it, "but as it was shark or fast he tried some." On another occasion, after going hungry for several days Elder Wood recorded: "We didn't have a thing in the house for breakfast this morning before prayer, but immediately after prayer, we had some fish and crackers brought to us, and by dinner time we had quite a bit of kalo brought in...."

After our usual breakfast of nothing and prayers we went out visiting.

All we had to eat today was a small breadfruit each, but the Lord made it sweet to our taste.[8]

Returning to the Saints on the mainland, we find an interesting assortment of fruits, nuts, and berries enjoyed by the Mormon people during the Nauvoo period of the Church. In the account book of merchant Amos Davis, we find mention made of "raisins to Wm. Felshaw," "Fayette apples to Oliver Gnanger," and "18 1/2 lbs. of almonds to Vinson Knight" among the grocery items.

If purchased by Latter-day Saints during the winter and spring of 1839-40, while the new settlement was still known by the old name of Commerce[9] *and in a letter written by William Clayton to Edward Martin, from Nauvoo, Illinois, November 29, 1840, the author rehearses encouraging things of a bright Nature: "The land is exceeding rich, wild grapes grow in great abundance. Also nuts of many kinds. Peaches, citrus, pumpkins, squashes, and good potatoes."*[10]

One did not need to live in Illinois in order to enjoy the "fruit of the land." Many Latter-day Saints residing elsewhere, had similar blessings. One old pioneer lady, recalling her childhood days in the South, fondly remembered what her family had to eat when they became converts to the Church:

Mary Raper Quin...was born on a plantation in Franklin County, Alabama...Always a lover of out of doors life, Mary spent much time wandering about the plantation. Mother

Nature seems to have been extra lavish to her children in the South. There were wild strawberries, gooseberries, huckleberries, peaches, scuppemongs, muskadines, persimmons, paw-paws, hickory nuts, walnuts, chestnuts, and pecans. No season of the year but what Mary and her sister could find something out in the woods to eat. She laughingly said the "Babes in the Woods" wouldn't have fared so badly in Alabama.[11]

Some fruit, though appealing in looks, could give more in the bite than a person had bargained for:

This is the forepart of October. It is warm and pleasant. I came to a tree filled with beautiful fruit, red on one side and yellow on the other. I was dry and hungry so I stepped up to the tree and picked some fruit and began to eat. It drew my face into all manner of shapes. I did not know what to make of it. I did not know but what the Lord wanted to make such fruit for. I thought it was something made in vain. I threw the fruit away and tried to straighten my face. I made all the attempts to do it but couldn't. Zebedee (Coltrin) laughed and made many expressions about me before the pucker left my mouth....

He told me the name of the fruit I had eaten some days back on the road that drew my mouth in such a shape. He said the fruit was good in its season and after the frosts came it would be good to eat. He called it "persimmon."[12]

After the Saints left the state of Illinois, they were deprived of many of the necessary fruits and vegetables which constitute a balanced nutrition. Because of this deficit in their diet, many of the people suffered severely from scurvy. However, things took a better turn for them when they temporarily stopped at Kanesville (Winter Quarters):

On the Iowa side of the river we raised wheat, Indian corn, buckwheat, potatoes, and other vegetables; and we gathered from the woods hazel and hickory nuts, white and black walnuts, and in addition to the wild plums and raspberries before mentioned, we gathered elderberries, and made elderberry and raspberry wine. We also preserved plums and berries. By these supplies we were better furnished than we had been since leaving our homes. The vegetables and FRUITS CAUSED THE SCURVY to pretty much DISAPPEAR.[13]

It is interesting to observe that once the Latter-day Saints were able to secure this natural food *THEIR RATE OF DISEASE DROPPED SIGNIFICANTLY.* And this because of the fruit they ate, for it acted as a cleansing agent upon their systems, thereby eliminating many impurities and sludgey matter gathered from long accumulation. It must be kept in mind that they had eaten a considerable amount of meat and starchy products prior this, which resulted in their weakened condition and subsequent illness thereafter. But now all of that seemed to be remedied with the introduction of healthier food items.

It could very well be that we, ourselves, might take a hint from all of this, and learn something from the pioneers. President Wilford Woodruff made the observation that Adam "was permitted to eat of the fruit of every tree except one."[14] To which Brigham Young wryly remarked about several months later: "If by eating one apple, Mother Eve ruined the whole human family, what would an orchard full of apples do?" And, in connection with this, we could well afford to ponder the question, "What would the general health of the Church be like if everyone ate *MORE FRUIT*, like the Saints at Winter Quarters did?' Perhaps an apple a day would keep more than just the doctor away, but also the source for all of our ill symptoms, with which we seem to be plagued so constantly.

During their historic trek across the barren wastelands of the Southwest, the famed Mormon Battalion suffered like privations of hunger and proper nourishment. However, upon their arrival in Santa Fe, New Mexico, they found "around the walks and in public places women and girls offering for sale, pine nuts, apples, peaches, large grapes, bread, onions, boiled corn, melons, etc."[16] To say the least, they took advantage of such delicacies and after eating trail dust and poor rations for so long, these new provisions seemed a God-send indeed.

When the Saints first arrived in the valleys, they had nothing much in the way of domestic fruit, save the wild mountain berries, currants, and certain kinds of grapes, which were scattered throughout the hills. Most of what came later had to be planted and developed. Hence, we find one pioneer sister writing to her children:

> *Now I will express a wish to my son Abiel Abbott, I want him to come down, and if he comes with a wagon, I wish him to bring some gooseberry bushes, some cherry trees, and some states currants, some blackberries, red and black raspberries and also apricot, prune, plum, nectarine and pear trees, also some peppermint...and some sand cherries...I think one can take small trees and box them up in dirt to bring them here. I want my*

lot filled with fruit trees and lucerne.[17]

By the early 1860s, the Mormon people had been fairly successful in their efforts to raise the things here which were lacking when they first came. A famous explorer of that time, Sir Richard Burton, paid a social visit to the "City of the Saints," and records the excellent products of Nature, which he found growing in the valley then:

A vineyard is now being planted on the hillside near Mr. Brigham Young's block, and homemade wine will soon become an item of produce in Utah. Pomology is carefully cultivated; about one hundred varieties of apples have been imported, and of these ninety-one are found to thrive as seedlings; in good seasons their branches are bowed down down by fruit, and must be propped up, or they will break under their load. The peaches were in all cases unpruned... Besides grapes and apples, there were walnuts, apricots and quinces, cherries and plums, currants, raspberries and gooseberries.[18]

There is even a mention of some fig trees being discovered in the Gentile mining town of Stockton, by one weary traveller.[19]

Despite the extensiveness of orchards and vineyards among the Saints, yet there were certain areas that were not as fortunately blessed as others were, and where the people often had to do without. One such place was the little Mormon community of St. Johns, Arizona. An early native recalls:

Fruit was a luxury there in those days. Only on rare and very special occasions were bananas and oranges brought in from the railroad, about sixty miles away. As soon as she could, she had an orchard and different berry bushes, using every inch of space that she had. Like it was yesterday, I remember the early peach tree that had ripe peaches in July. Oh, how eagerly we watched them get ripe. It seemed like they would never ripen and how good they were. The first fruit that they "put up" there for winter was put in cans with a tin lid soldered on with some kind of rosin. They "dried" fruit for winter and found it quite satisfactory, and when they had glass bottles that seemed just perfect. Now we have frozen fruits. What development!

But as the people of God prospered, so did their pride and vanity. Abundance brought with it a carelessness for the bounty of the earth, and the generous harvest soon seen part of the bumper crop rotting around the trees as next year's compost:

> *This was the period in Utah's early history when wives and daughters were glad to have wool, which they could manufacture into clothing for themselves and families, in which we were all so comfortable and so proud. But these days passed, when through want of food in early spring time the sego, the thistle top, and the famine root, were sought as food and more relished and enjoyed than now, in all that wealth can produce. And while it was with nimble feet, and in such cheerful and loving companionship that we, of all ages, could trip away to the canyon or mountain sides for the service-berry, the wild raspberry, currant and choke cherry. All of these we then considered luscious, but now they were forgotten, while the apple, pear, peach and plum, and other choice FRUITS ARE IN SUCH WASTEFUL ABUNDANCE. But in this surfeit of blessings, have our hearts continued to feel the same gratitude to God and the same love for each other?*[21]

These observations were made by Benjamin F. Johnson and it would do well for some of us to reflect about them in our own time, and realize just how important they are.

Nuts have played an important role in the Mormon diet, too. One lady fondly recalls her pioneer childhood days of yesteryear:

> *One thing we did that was fun was the pine nut hunts. When the pine nuts were ripe all the young folks on the Creek and some of the Indians would all get together and burn the trees that had the nuts on. Of course, the green trees did not burn much, but it would heat the cones that held the nuts so they would fall. Sometimes they would cut the tree down and cover it with earth, then make a fire on top of the earth. In this way the nuts could be roasted and the cones would open easily.*[22]

Sister Leah D. Widstoe had this to say about the nutritional value in nuts:

> *Nuts are one of Nature's most nourishing foods, for they are rich in protein and precious vitamins, especially in vitamin B, as well as food minerals. While lean meat contains 15% to 19% protein, nuts contain 21% to 25% protein. Hence, nuts may be considered as essentially a protein food, and they should be so used in the dietary. Yet the protein of nuts is not as easily*

digested as meat protein, partly because of the difficulty of mastication. This too should be a guide to their use. As an occasional substitute for meat, nuts are valuable, though they should be prepared in such a way that they may be well masticated and should not be fed to small children unless they are taught to chew thoroughly.[23]

In reaching a concluding summary on the material presented herein, the following is offered as proof of our lack of good nutrition:

To improve our physical standard, the first thing to do is to awaken the interest of the public in the matter. It is necessary to show that, although we are the same race, with the same climate and the same water that we had, say 120 years ago, WE HAVE PHYSICALLY DETERIORATED—the reason being that our diet has changed during that time.

What is the remedy, the cure for this appalling condition?

Eat grains, vegetables and FRUITS OF THE EARTH—as FRESH as they may possibly be secured and as nearly as may be possible in that consumption![24]

Recent evidence seems to indicate that in a few areas of Utah the people are becoming more consciously aware of the fact that proper diet is an important thing to have in order that good health may constantly be maintained. Over the television news of Friday, February 13, 1976, a Salt Lake TV station announced at their noonday broadcast that the Provo School Board has banned the sale of all artificial sweets and candies for a period of six months. The report also made mention of unhappy comments from the various schools in the district over this new ruling. The critics claimed that such a move seriously curtailed badly needed revenues obtained from these sales, to fund special school projects with. Despite this mild opposition, the decision remained as originally given.

What was significant about the whole is that a proposal was made and adopted to sell milk, *FRUIT AND OTHER NATURAL SWEETS* in the schools, in place of the candies. The entire action was a result of massive campaigning on the part of the Provo Dental Association. The new program will continue on a trial basis, for the next sixteen weeks.

There can be no doubt whatsoever that a faithful diet of natural fruit will invariably guarantee one good health and eventually insure prolonged longevity. Positive proof of such results may be seen in the remarkable life span of the late President Joseph Fielding Smith. While others his age and younger were crippled with this malady or stricken with that affliction, he continued to "blossom as the rose" long after the others had wilted and faded away. At the astonishing age of 93, he became head of one of the most successful and busy organizations upon the face of the earth today—namely, the Church of Jesus Christ of Latter-day Saints—and seemed to function quite well in his new capacity, despite the advanced years against him.

What was the secret of his "eternal youth"? It may lay in a statement his wife, Jessie Evans Smith, made six years ago in April: "My husband doesn't eat meat. *WE EAT LOTS OF FRUITS AND VEGETABLES!"*[25] What finer testimony would a person need than this, to convince him that "living like Crusoe" is the only way to go, in order to be assured of sounder, physical health, greater peace of mind, and a brighter tomorrow, free from the debilitating factors which now ravage the human system.

Now Robinson Crusoe lived a ripe, old age,
And turned each day of his life as a page;
For more than a volume or single book,
Would contain the things his mortality took.

Upon his death-bed, all wizened and gray,
Friday pleaded in earnest, "Oh tell me I pray—
The secret of life to your extended youth;
For I wish to know such, now tell me the truth."

Old Crusoe, he raised himself up and said,
"Now get this through your thick savage head:
You know these years the mangoes and oranges I've tried?"
("Yessire")—"Well, they're my secret to life on this side!"

NOTES

1. John Heinerinan, "Poems and Verse," unpublished manuscript, Manti, Utah.

2. Journals of Elder C. J. Hansen, Harold B. Lee Library, BYU, Provo, Utah. Ledger Book for March 30, 1899 entry. *1899 Missionary Journal*: pp. 30-31 (March 31, 1899); p. 36 (April 14th entry); pp. 40—41, (May 1, 1899); p. 43 (May 7th); p. 44 (May 9th); p. 53 (June 17th); pp. 55—56 (July 4th); pp. 58—59 (July 14th); p. 60 (July 17th); p. 61 (July 20th); p. 62 (July 26); p.63 (August 4th); p. 64 (August 7th); p, 65 (August 16th); p. 70 (September 11th); p. 71 (September 15th); p. 74 (September 29th); p. 76 (October 7th); p. 81 (October 23rd); pp. 86-87 (November 24th); p. 88 (December 2nd); p. 88 (December 3rd); p. 88 (December 4th); *1900 Missionary Journal* pp. 1 (January lst); pp. 5-6 (January 9th); p. 7 (January 13th); p. 10 (January 23rd); p. 22 (April l8th); p. 27 (May 23rd) ; pp. 28—29 (May 25—26, 27, 28, 29); p. 36 (June 17th) ; p. 38 (June 18 & 20); p.41 (June 28th); pp. 42—43 (July 4th); pp. 43—4 4 (July 5th); p. 49 (August 6th); p. 50 (August 8th); p. 54 (August 21st); p. 55 (August 24th); pp. 56- 57 (August 27th & 28th); p. 65 (October 18th); p. 66 (October 23rd); p. 67 (November 1—5, 1900); pp. 76-77 (January 15, 1901); p. 76 (February 14-20, 1901), *1901 Missionary Journal*: p. 1 (September 23rd-October 5th); p. 5 (January 1st, 1902).

3. George Q. Cannon, *My First Mission—The First Book of The Faith-Promoting Series*; Salt Lake, 1882, pp. 33—34.

4. *Ibid.*, pp. 33, 61.

5. Eliza R. Snow Smith, *Biography and Family Record of Lorenzo Snow*; Salt Lake, 1884, p. 431.

6. Cannon, *op., cit.*, pp. 32-33.

7. Augusta Joyce Crocheron, *Representative Women of Deseret*; Salt Lake, 1884, p. 79.

8. Melvin S. Tagg, *The Life of Edward James Wood, Church Patriot;* July, 1959, pp. 25-49. Unpublished thesis at Harold B. Lee Library, BYU, Provo.

9. Amos Davis Account Book, *op., cit.*

10. Kate B. Carter, Historical Pamphlet, December, 1943; "Pioneer Letters of Historical Value"; p. 379.

11. Roberta Clayton, *op., cit.*, Mary R, Quinn History, fd. #131, bx. 2.

12. *Diary of Levi W. Hancock*, pp. 60, 62. Typescript copy in possession of the author.

13. Edward Tullidge, *The Women of Mormondom*; New York, 1877, p. 341.

14. *JD* 15:78.

15. *Deseret Weekly* 21:440, August 18, 1872.

16. Journal History, October 10, 1846, *op., cit.*

17. Carter, Historical Pamphlet, *op., cit.*, p, 403.

18. Richard F. Burton, *The City of the Saints*; New York, 1862, pp. 269—270.

19. John Codman, *The Round Trip*; New York, 1879, p. 184.

20. "My Pioneer Grandmother—Anna Dorthea J. Kempe," 'Roberta Clayton Collection, *op., cit.*, p. 6; fd. #79, bx. 1.

21. Benjamin F. Johnson, *My Life's Review*; Independence, 1947; p.201.

22. "Pine Valley Days," by Julia Putnam Foster; Utah Humanities Foundation, Marriott Library, University of Utah, Salt Lake City.

23. Leah D. Widstoe, *op., cit.*, p,. 258.

24. *Millennial Star*, 93:137—138.

25. *Era* 73:59, April, 1970.

CHAPTER SEVEN

THE VIRTUES IN DESERET

(Honey, Molasses, Sorghum, and Sugar—Pioneer Staples)

"And they did also carry with them deseret, which, by interpretation, is a honey bee..."[1] Thus did the Jaredites bring with them one of the most important substances known to man and one of the most natural foods available—honey—when they settled these two great continents of North and South America.

But honey is not a new introduction to civilization. It is as old as man and the scriptures themselves. Great men of God in ages past have received their sustenance and strength from this natural product. "And the same John had [as] his food...locusts and wild honey."[2]

Now as to touching the item of "locusts." It has always been thought by many that this which John the Baptist ate in the wilderness was insect-like grasshoppers. Nothing could be further from the truth. "Locusts" are a special kind of tree commonly found in Palestine. Another name for it is the carob tree. Its leaves are like those of our ash, but the leaflets more rounded, and very dark glossy, and evergreen. It blossoms at the end of February, and the pods are found in enormous quantities in April and May. They are flat and narrow, from six to ten inches in length, of the shape of a horn—whence the Greek name. Before they are ripe they are agreeable and sweetish when chewed, reminding one somewhat of the pods of the tamarind in the West Indies, and, like that fruit, are often used steeped in water to supply a pleasant and cooling drink.

In the famous parable of the prodigal son, the Master used the "husks" of this tree to illustrate the most abject poverty to which one may be reduced, both materially as well as spiritually, if he leaves that which is good and turns to a life of wasteful living. These husks are to be seen on the stalls in all Oriental towns, where they are sold for food, but are chiefly used for the feeding of cattle and horses, and especially for pigs. Such is what the disobedient son was finally reduced to, having to content himself with the unsatisfying remains of the carob plant as a symbol of this world's enjoyment.[3]

Such an explanation may not seem very credulous in the light of that which is too often easily based upon mere assumption alone. Yet such is what the Prophet John ate in his time. And another Man of God, almost nineteen hundred years later, partook of the very same things. The second was none other than Elder Lorenzo Snow. In 1872 President Brigham Young called upon the apostle to select some suitable individual who could be able to accompany him to the Holy Land. Brother Snow and his party commenced their journey shortly thereafter, and eventually reached their destination sometime in the early winter of 1973. Of course, winter to them over there was comparable to an Indian summer here. During his stay in the land of the nativity, he had occasion to eat a variety of things, among which was included the customary Carob and some delicious wild honey from the regions thereabout. Thus did Apostle Snow share in the same delightful foods of Nature, which John himself had been permitted to do, so long ago.[4]

Honey is a very delicious item, and as such one would think it would satisfy the appetites of ordinary men. Yet something so pleasant as this cannot always help to sweeten the surly disposition of human nature. During the march of Zion's Camp to the land of Independence for the purpose of "redeeming Zion," "most of the men in the camp complained to Joseph Smith of sore toes, blistered feet, long drives, scanty supply of provisions, poor quality of bread, bad corndodger, frouzy butter, maggoty bacon and cheese, *AND STRONG HONEY*! Even a dog could not bark at some of the men without their murmuring..."

Imagine this, if you will—complaints of "strong honey"—as if the bees should have known better to make it milder. The audacity of some people is outrageous, and when one considers the times that many have been in want of some nourishing substance to sustain them, it is with a sad and heavy heart that one shakes his head at such deplorable conduct on the part of priesthood brethren. As Elder George A. Smith put it: "...we were the Camp of Zion, and many of us were heedless, foolish or devilish, and yet we did not know it. Joseph had to bear with us and tutor us like children. There were many, however, in the Camp, who never murmured and were always ready and willing to do as our leader desired."[6]

The Saints would often gather their honey from the forest, as did Elder Jonathan Dunham, during the Nauvoo period of 1843: "Monday 8—Went about eight or ten miles after wild honey; found two trees, got the honey, and returned home by dark the same day."[7]

It seems that the early pioneers relied upon this substance more in the wild than they did in a domestic sense. Careful research has failed to turn up any plausible evidence to support the theory that they might have attempted to raise their own. In fact, an abundance of information seems to indicate just the contrary—that they secured it in the same manner which Elder Dunham had done his.

The Mormon people had ingenious ways of locating wild hives, and surprising methods of storing the honey afterwards.

> *One day Mr. Barton saw some bees gathered around the waterhole. Now he was a natural bee-man. He knew there must be some hollow trees not far where they stored their honey. He fixed up some sugar and water into a syrup and put the plate containing it where they could find it—then with a handful of flour, he waited. Soon the bees found the syrup and he managed to sprinkle them with the flour then watch which way they went. It was not long before he located three or four trees filled with honey.*
>
> *There was the honey all right, but what could he store it in? Deer were plentiful so he killed one, took the skin off whole by cutting it around the neck and just above the hooves of the four feet. The skin stretches very readily when it is wet, so he peeled it off, washed and dried it thoroughly, then made a bag of it by tying the leg opening with buckskin and using the neck through which to pour the honey. It served as an excellent storage receptacle, the honey keeping fresh and pure therein as long as it lasted.*
>
> *The venison was cut in strips and dried as "jerky" and was very choice eating. After the buckskin had served its purpose as a bag, it was cut up and used as moccasins for the boys and Mr. Barton to wear.*[8]

Not all were entirely successful in their ventures, especially if they became greedy and wanted to consume some right on the spot:

> *Wild honey was plentiful and it was not hard to follow the bees to their trees and get what honey we needed. One time Mr. Hough almost choked to death when he and my husband were robbing a bee-tree. He got a piece of large honey-comb stuck in his throat and had hard work to get it out.*[9]

So important was the matter of honey to the Latter-day Saints that it became permanently enshrined in their religion. The pioneer composer Evan Stevens lauded the virtues of Mormon children in search of truth, with a timely composition appropriately titled "The Bees of Deseret," in which the singers were the little winged creatures and knowledge was depicted as honey.

We are the bees of Deseret,
The busy, busy, cheerful bees,
Gathering what honey we can get
From all the flowers blooming on the trees;
Trying to fill our little hives
With every good that we can gather round;
Wisdom and truth, eternal lives.
These are the priceless treasures we have found.

CHORUS:

Workers are we, no idlers here
Shall live among our busy, happy band;
We gather honey all the year,
And plenty can be found on every hand

Like other bees, we love to sing,
Our voices ever sounding sweet and clear,
And all the valley often ring
With happy, cheerful songs we love so dear.
We still will labor with our might;
While yet 'tis day, to gather wisdom strive,
That when the night comes we'll have light,
Eternal light to shine within our hives.[10]

The state symbol became the beehive, and adorned many buildings and public works in the territorial days. Evidence of this unique heritage still remains in our time. The entrance to the Utah State Fairgrounds is majestically capped with an enormous beehive, and several little "bees of Deseret" in the act of crawling around on top. Highway patrol cars have the insignia emblazoned upon the doors of their vehicles. In fact, Utah has come to be known as "The Beehive State." Not for the honey we produce, but for what the pioneers left us with.

It seems, though, that molasses constituted a greater part of the Mormon diet than did honey. References are more numerous and occasions more frequent wherein this substance was used in place of the latter. The first settlers to southern Utah relied quite heavily upon "bread and molasses and beef and squash"[11] for their main staples.

Molasses was obtained in various ways, from different sources.

> *During that year quite a variety of good vegetables was raised. The melons, pumpkin and squash were very sweet. I made corn stalk molasses in my wash boiler...I thought I had never eaten anything so good.*[12]

Preparation of this commodity was a big thing in those days. It rivaled the familiar "husking bees" of the Midwest.

> *The first move of the family...was from Toquerville to Virgin City, Utah (1854)... They raised cane and made their own molasses. When the molasses season was ending, they would cut up their fruit, put it in the vats where the molasses was made and make their preserves. Oftentimes all the women in the town would join on the occasions, and thus the molasses and preserving seasons were made into a regular sort of holiday.*[13]

Another reminisced: "Molasses time was another big time for us. Most of the families made their molasses together and we would have a candy pulling after the molasses was cooked."[14]

And a third remembered: "We had honey, taffy, and molasses candy...and a huge can or jar filled with molasses cookies, a custom I have kept up to this day... Father liked simple wholesome foods and was usually very frugal."[15]

However, these favorite 'candy pulls' were not always enjoyable for some. Things could get out-of-hand and rather sticky at times:

> *Mother had gone to the nearest store. It took her three days to make the trip. She left me to care for the family and told me to have the house all cleaned when she came back. She had one treasure, a rocking chair, the only one in the country round, and she never left the house without warning us to be careful of it.*
>
> *The third day came and I scrubbed and scoured everything, blackened the stove until you could see your face in it. Fixed what we had in the house for supper—she would bring a fresh supply—and waited for her to come. When bedtime came I went to bed, tired out but happy because everything looked so nice and Mother would be pleased.*

I had only retired when here came my brother from Choir practice, and with him all the young people of the neighborhood. They made some molasses candy, played "snatch grab" with it, wrapped it around the girls necks and tangled it in each other's hair. It had boiled over and burned on my polished stove, and soon it was all over everything in the house, but the worst was yet to come—they broke the prized rocking chair. At last they were gone, but I was too tired to get up and clean the house again. I might as well have done as I could not sleep for thinking of the chair kept me awake. As soon as... [rest of page was typed over twice, thereby making it illegible to read].[16]

Obviously, a licking resulted and it was *NOT* someone's tongue at the end of a molasses spoon, either!

In those days, when tithing was paid in kind, wages for labor performed was also imparted in a similar manner: "We went out to Holladay and lived in a little adobe room a few weeks and Father got a job working at a molasses mill. He got molasses for pay."[17]

Molasses candy was one of the big surprises at Christmas time. Children seemed satisfied with so little then, and this nourishing treat went a long way to make many little Saints very happy.

Alma Chambers remarked: "Christmas in the early days was very different from what it is today. There were no gifts, only candy. This was usually homemade molasses, or stick candy.

Another pioneer says: "On Christmas we never had a tree and we did not receive so many beautiful gifts. It was just the spirit of the day that made everything so nice. We would hang up our stockings and get an apple and maybe some (molasses) candy in it."

Levi Edgar Young wrote: "But in those far-gone days, the children were taught to appreciate any little gift. There was no store full of toys, as we have them today. The gift was always an expression of the great love of the giver. Sometimes a man gave a beaver skin or buffalo robe to his wife and children. The gift made them all happy. Often the head of a household provided venison and wild fowl for a feast, and all shared and neighbors were invited to partake. There was no selfishness; no envy; no bigotry. People did not hold themselves aloof from others. There was social equality, and a regard for one another that was sincere!

Children did not have every whim satisfied; they were pleased with any little plaything and the dissatisfaction seen around the young people today was absent from the home and school.[18]

The value of molasses in our time cannot be discredited. Any sensible person knows that such a natural food as this is wonderful for the body and provides strength and energy which other products of its type do not. However, some from the sophist school of modern thought feel otherwise, and by their eloquence and educated charm seek to mislead the people with a careful juggling of the facts:

Blackstrap molasses is another controversial food. There are advocates of black-strap molasses who have stated that it is rich in iron and copper. Most of the copper is due to contamination of the blackstrap at the food processing plant, that is, from the containers and pipes through which it flows when it is processed. It was represented as effective in B vitamin deficiency. Sufficient medical evidence has never been forth coming to justify these extravagant claims.[19]

Despite these clever insinuations, the proper worth of molasses was highlighted by Sister Leah D. Widstoe:

It may be said that old-fashioned molasses is a valuable "sweet," for it contains not only its carbohydrate value, but some protein, phosphorus, and definite amounts of calcium, iron, and manganese. Blackstrap molasses is AN EXCELLENT SOURCE OF VALUABLE MINERALS and contains as well most of the vitamins of the B complex, with the exception of thiamin (Bl). There is much to be said in favor of the old-fashioned pioneer dessert of whole wheat bread and molasses.

The iron in molasses is high enough to deserve investigation as to its efficiency in nutrition. Hard molasses cookies, especially when made with whole wheat flour or with part of the wheat flour replaced by rolled oats, would seem to be an excellent sweet for children, if used in moderation at the end of a meal.[20]

Sorghum also played an important part in the Mormon diet. Most of this crop was grown in southern Utah. An excerpt from a song describing the hardships of pioneers settling in St. George goes:

My wagon sold for sorghum seed to make a little bread,
And poor old Jim and Bally both long ago are dead.
There's only me and Betsy left to hoe the cotton tree,
May Heaven help the Dixieite, wherever he may be.[21]

It formed one of the basic staples which settlers came to rely on quite a bit for food:

A day for my parents was from daylight until dark—all work. They produced most of what we had. For the first few years we lived on cornbread (cornmeal mush for night) with plenty of good milk, butter, most kinds of vegetables and sorghum. We seemed to strive and do well.[22]

Among the food items covered in this chapter, none seemed to be in such scarce a supply as sugar. Emily Dow Partridge Young remembered that after her father, Bishop Edward Partridge, and his family were driven from Jackson County, Missouri in 1832, he "left what provisions he had, in his house. I do not remember of there being more than one pound of sugar in our house at a time until I left home. Father used to buy it by the barrel...but he gave it all for the gospel's sake."[23]

Furthermore, her father recommended that Latter day Saint mothers should not give their children any sweets, or "sugar cookies" as he referred to them, after they have punished their youngsters for an act of disobedience. He said that all too often mothers were inclined to feel sorry for their "precious, little dears," and seek to win back their favor or stop them from crying by enticing them with some type of a sweet. He emphasized that this was terribly wrong to do—that a child justly punished should not in any way be shown special favor or consideration afterwards, but allowed to be left alone so that he or she could learn the lesson well for which they were disciplined.[24]

Henry William Bigler recalls how they obtained sugar in Harrison County, West Virginia, at the time he joined the Church in 1837:

The last of February and the first of March was the time for making sugar from the sugar trees, and before the time came to open camp for making sugar, troughs were made and placed at the sugar trees and spiles already made, and when the time came for opening camp, the trees were tapped by boring auger holes and with a light mallet or hatchet, the piles were driven into the holes, the troughs holding from two to three gallons of sugar water. The kettles kept boiling day and night, when there was a good run of sugar water and every day sugar was made from 10, 20 and 30 pounds of sugar made every day ascending to the supply of water from the sugar trees. At such times everybody who happened to be present, children and all was made welcome to eat all the new sugar they wished. I was delighted when sugar-making time came, although it was hard work to gather sugar water when there was a good run and to keep the kettles (3, 4 and 5) boiling which was done day and night. [24a]

The availability of sugar in Nauvoo seems to have been rather plentiful, for the store accounts of various regular customers reveals that grocer Amos Davis was able to meet both supply and demand of the same in a very able manner.

But in the Utah period things seemed to be a bit different. Horace Greeley made this observation while visiting the territory in the 1850s:

"Sugar is another necessary of life which they have had bad luck with. They can grow the beet very well, but it is said to yield little or no sugar—because, it is supposed, of an excess of alkali in the soil. The sorghum has not yet been turned to much account, but it is to be. Common brown sugar sells here at sixty cents per pound..."[25]

As sugar became harder to find, the price went higher.

Our sugar was all gone, but about this time a man brought some in from California. I had waited with others for an hour and a half to get into the house where it was, and then could only have one pound of brown sugar, for which I paid one dollar.[26]

With this kind of inflation around, the more resourceful turned to devising other means as a substitution for such an expensive item:

One winter before the sugar factories were brought into that valley [Utah County], sugar and honey were scarce, but they had had a bounteous harvest of squash. Freezing the squash turned the liquid very sweet, so she and her mother cut squashes and put them out on the snow to freeze. Then they put them in pans in the house to thaw. The juice which drained from them was boiled to a syrup and this was used to sweeten their pies, pumpkin butter, which was used as a spread for their bread, and other desserts.[27]

During this critical period of little product and outrageous prices, a wonderful thing took place with many of the Saints in Utah, which equalled, if not surpassed, the miracle of the "manna from heaven" with the Children of Israel in olden times. It was the day everyone would remember as a special act of divine providence, when "sugar from the Lord" came in a mysterious way.

"The Spring of 1855 opened under more favorable circumstances; still many of the Saints went without the comforts of life. Provisions were very high. Sugar, for instance, was worth a dollar a pound in Provo. In August, 1855, a memorable blessing was given to the people of Provo in the shape of a hard, white substance found upon the leaves of young cottonwood trees. We shook this substance, which was very sweet, into tubs of water and boiled it down without process, when it congealed into sugar about the color of our common brown sugar. The Saints in Provo made between three and four thousand pounds of this kind of sugar. I told the Saints that it was a direct gift from the Lord and they freely paid their tithing on it. Among other products, I took three hundred thirty-three pounds of this sugar to Salt Lake City to the general tithing office. On explaining the matter to President Brigham Young, whom I met at the door, he declared it was 'sugar from the Lord.'" (Elias H. Blackburn)

George Washington Adam relates the following: He and his family were moving to St. George to raise cotton. They traveled as far as Provo, where they visited with the family of George A. Smith, and helped to gather leaves for the purpose of making sugar and syrup. They would gather the leaves, wash them in tubs, strain the water and boil down to form sugar or syrup. He took quite a supply with him to Dixie.

Mrs. Emmeline Baldwin, of Monroe, Sevier County, records the following in a history written by herself: "I remember in the early fifties, there was a white substance which came on the leaves of cottonwood and willow trees. It was sweet and people went and camped on the Provo River bottoms, where it was abundant, to gather it. They would break off the branches, wash off the substance in a vessel of water, strain it, and then boil it down. The sugar obtained was similar to maple sugar. It was put into pans, where it hardened into cakes."[28]

And Julia S. Ferrin recalls in her mother's life:

"It was also in this time that the Lord provided sugar in the form of a white sticky substance that came overnight on all of the shrubs and bushes around. The people broke off the bushes or limbs and dipped them in water. Then they made a sweet syrup by boiling it down. They used this in place of sugar. My mother learned to depend on the Lord in her early girlhood and she never let her faith die. Even in her old age she relied upon the Lord and asked special blessings.[29]

Raw sugar from the natural source is what the pioneers used. Its nutritional benefits can never be dismissed as minimal. But again, there are those in our midst who would have us think otherwise: "...the amounts of vitamins and minerals found in raw sugar are infinitesimal, and we obtain plenty of them in a normal well-balanced diet."[30]

Leah D. Widstoe said that "white sugar...is *NOT* a natural food product, but is made artificially, and in the process the juice of the cane or beet is robbed of all its possible mineral content and not only is the product treated by bleaching gases, but it is blued to give it a dead white color."[3]

It should be kept in mind that children love sweets. All ages, all sizes, are susceptible to the magic of a treat.

Julia was very fond of pine gum. The morning they were to start home, she left camp with several others in search of a little more pine gum. As it took the men folks quite awhile to tend their teams, pack their wagons and get ready to leave, she felt that there was plenty of time to go a little farther from camp where she could select some choice pieces of gum. The farther she went the better the gum seemed to be. She became so engrossed she failed to notice that her companions had left one by one. She heard shouting and thinking they were perhaps getting ready to leave, started running as she thought, towards camp.

Presently, she could hear wagons moving and she ran faster and faster, but no camp was in sight. When she became exhausted from running, she became frightened and began to realize that she must be lost. Although she was panic-stricken, she had presence of mind enough to stop running and to try to get her bearings. She could no longer hear shouting or the moving of wagons. As she stood there, scanning the countryside she saw in the distance what she thought to be a moving wagon, so she started running in that direction; if it were a wagon there surely must be a road which would help her to find her way. When she found the road, another wagon came along which directed her to camp. Although many busy years passed since that day, Julia never forgot the terrible feeling of being lost in the forest.[32]

In conclusion, we should keep in mind what Apostle John A. Widstoe said about the use of sweet foods in our diet:

> *The body needs sugar; it is a physiological necessity, for it is found as glucose in the blood (about one part to one thousand) and provides fuel for heat and muscular energy... Even Nature's sweet foods, fresh or dried fruits, honey or syrup (molasses), are good foods, but their proper use should be understood and followed; they should be eaten MODERATELY, usually as a dessert.*
>
> *There are many disadvantages resulting from the excessive use of sugar as food. It is distinctly a habit-forming food; those who have never used it do not like it, but a taste for it is easily acquired, after which one is tempted to overeat on sweet foods which leads to an unbalanced diet. This habit-forming Nature has contributed greatly to the consumption of sugar.*[33]

For ourselves, for our children, and for our health, we should keep these things in mind, and realize that even though there is a distinct advantage to using the natural products in Nature for our food, such as honey, molasses, sorghum, and brown sugar, it should be kept in mind that discretion is needed and good, sound judgment applied in the amount of consumption pertaining to each item. After all, we wouldn't want to get lost in the woods like the little girl with the pine gum, and never be able to find our way back to good health—now would we?

NOTES

1. Ether 2:3.
2. Matthew 3:30.
3. H.B. Tristram, *The Natural History of the Bible*; London, 1868, pp. 360-362.
4. For further information in regards to Elder Snow's delightful trip, please consult the supplement section in the back of "Biography and Family Record of Lorenzo Snow" by Eliza R. Snow Smith, pp. 542—558, comprising Letters VII - X.
5. *Contributor* 4:45.
6. *Ibid.*
7. *DHC* 5:545.
8. " "Elizabeth A. Greenshaw," Roberta Clayton, *op., cit.*, fd. #50, bx. #1.
9. "Autobiography of Rosetta Schmutz Hunt," *Ibid.*, fd. #66, bx. #1.
10. *Deseret Sunday School Songs*, 1909, p. 42.
11. William Mulder and A. Russell Mortensen, *Among The Mormons*; Lincoln, 1958, p. 432.
12. Preston Nibley, *op., cit.*, p. 69 (Cited previously elsewhere).
13. "Rosilpha S. Gardner," Roberta Clayton, *op., cit.*, fd. #45, bx. #1.
14. "Pine Valley Days" by Julia Putnam Foster; Utah Humanities Foundation, Marriott Library, University of Utah, Salt Lake City.
15. Kate B. Carter, "Pioneer Celebrations," Historical Pamphlet, December 1939; p. 8.
16. "Annie C. H. Whipple," Roberta Clayton, *op., cit.*, fd. #184, bx #4.
17. "Ten Autobiographies," Andrew Hansen. Kate B. Carter, *Our Pioneer Heritage*, p. 68.
18. Milton R. Hunter, *Beneath Ben Lomond's Peak*; p. 125.

19. Leadership Week, David D. Geddes, *op., cit.*, p. 18. (Previously cited).

20. Leah B. Widstoe, *op., cit.*, p. 95.

21. George A. Flicks; "Folklore of Washington County, Utah," by Maralyn Winson, p. 15. Utah Humanities Foundation, Marriott Library, University of Utah, Salt Lake City.

22. "Autobiography of John Lowe Sevy," p. 3. Utah Humanities Foundation, *Ibid.*

23. "Diary of Emily Dow Partridge Young," December 1876, p. 22, BYU, Provo.

24. *Ibid.*

24a. Journal of Henry William Bigler.

25. Horace Greeley, *An Overland Journey*; New York, 1964, p. 199.

26. Preston Nibicy, *op., cit.*, p. 70.

27. Harriet A. Duff; Roberta Clayton, *op., cit.*, fd. #20, bx. #1.

28. Kate B. Carter, *Heart Throbs of the West*; Salt Lake, 1941, Volume 3, p. 360.

29. "A Short History of My Mother's Life (Elizabeth Clark McBride)" by Julia E. Ferrin; Roberta Clayton Collection, *op., cit.*, p. 2, fd. #95, bx. #2.

30. David B. Geddes, *op., cit.*, p. 18.

31. Leah B. Widstoe, *op., cit.*, pp. 94-95.

32. "Julia Smith Ballard," Roberta Clayton, *op., cit.*, fd. #4, bx. #1.

33. Widstoe's Word of Wisdom, *op., cit.*, p. 180.

CHAPTER EIGHT

OIL IN THEIR VESSELS

(Joseph Smith and Consecrated Olive Oil)

"They that were foolish took no oil; but the wise took oil in their vessels."[1] So said the Savior in his famous parable of the ten virgins. The allusion which he gave to the word "vessel" here is the same type of one which the Apostle Paul gave in his epistle to the Thessalonians some years later: "Every one of you should know how to possess his vessel in sanctification and honor."[2] In both instances it was given to mean the mortal tabernacle of man.

In the early days of the Church a peculiar custom prevailed among the first Latter-day Saints. It was the habit of taking natural olive oil internally as a form of medicine or healing remedy for a specific ailment. It was also used externally upon many afflicted parts of the body as a type of "balm of Gilead." This practice was first introduced into the Mormon faith by the Prophet Joseph Smith:

> *My father, William P. McIntire, lived in Nauvoo, on the corner of Main and Parley streets. He was a near neighbor to the Prophet, and a true and loving watch-guard for him in times of trouble.*
>
> *The Prophet Joseph was often at my father's house. One morning when he called at our house, I had a very sore throat. It was much swollen and gave me great pain. He took me up in his lap, and gently anointed my throat with consecrated oil and administered to me, and I was healed. I had no more pain nor soreness.* [3]

This natural product of great value was oil which had been formally blessed by the Elders of the Church in a simple ceremony involving the Melchizedek Priesthood. It was their belief that by invoking the Spirit of God, divine power would be allowed to pass through the liquid held in their hands, thus sanctifying the elements therein, making it a holy and consecrated substance of the purest sort. And once this had been touched by the "finger of the Lord," it would work miraculous benefits of great healing for them who had faith in such things.

Now, Joseph Smith believed in this with all of his heart and soul, and taught the higher priesthood the importance of its constant use when occasion would require it. Having learned their lessons well from such a great man, the members were able to test the strength of his remarks later on and prove to themelves that what he had said about its internal and external use was all correct and valid:

> *On November 12, 1844...I was directed to go to the house of Brother David Smith and administer to him, his wife and sister, as they were all very sick with the chills and fever (commonly called "the shakes")...*
>
> *Brother David lay upon a bed in one corner and his wife, Phoebe upon another. She whispered, "Bless me." She was shaking harder, if possible, than Sister Lucy had done. I never came so near saying, "I cannot," during my life since. The voice in my ear, with that sarcastic "Ha! ha!" said: "You can do no more, you are a fool and can do nothing." At this stage life and light seemed to enter me. I took the oil and anointed her head and sealed it upon her and commanded her to cease shaking and be made whole. From that moment she ceased shaking.*
>
> *Upon glancing around, I discovered Sister Lucy dressed and building a fire to cook some food. I turned to Brother David. He reached my hand and placed it upon his head. It seemed to me that no man could shake as he did. That voice said, "You need not try him for you cannot stop him." I took the oil in my hand and said, "Satan close they mouth." I GAVE Brother David A SPOONFULL OF OIL and I fairly poured the oil over his head and anointed his neck and shoulders and sealed the same, commanding him in the authority of the Holy Priesthood to cease shaking and be made whole, and telling the adversary, in the name of the Lord, to leave the house.*
>
> *How long I wrestled I know not, but I know that most of the afternoon had slipped away and the shadows of evening were gathering around. The family were healed and I know it was by the power of God. From that day to this I have never had a doubt. To the Almighty be all the honor.*

Besides serving as a remedy for severe fevers, consecrated olive oil was also an excellent antidote for deadly poisons taken into the system unawares:

> *Another very remarkable case of prophecy and healing came under my observation the following spring. A revelation was given by the Spirit, in tongues, to the effect that one of our number would be poisoned by the enemies of the Church, and be brought nigh to death, but that if she was faithful and sent for the Elders of the Church, she should be restored.*
>
> *This warning was repeated twice at intervals of about a month. On the last occasion, in addition, it was stated that the person giving the interpretation would be the sufferer. This terrible idea so affected her that she was completely, overcome. After recovering, she proceeded home, and the weather being warm, she drank some sweetened water, which she had prepared in the morning, and had left in an exposed situation, for use. When she had done this the second time, she felt her mouth burn. She immediately declared she was poisoned, and commenced retching violently until she became blind. Her husband, after procuring a person to stay with her, left for one of the Elders, but as he had to go some six miles before he returned with myself, she was, to all appearance, dead, and had not been perceived to breathe for an hour. Upon arriving at the house, I asked the Lord to cause her to breathe, if she was to recover. Upon looking at her closely, I perceived that she gave two distinct gasps, such as are usually given when the breath is leaving the body. Had I not seen this, I should have concluded that she was dead, for the women who were watching with her said, directly we entered, that she was dead, and had been so an hour. I then administered unto her in the name of Jesus, and prayed the Lord to preserve her life till my son-in-law returned with some oil which he had gone to procure. As soon as I had done this, she was able to speak sufficiently, in a "whisper," to ask for some water, but, so great was her weakness, she fell over on her face when raised to receive the water. The oil arriving, WE ADMINISTERED SOME TO HER INTERNALLY, in the name of the Lord, when she arose without any assistance, saying, "I am healed. I am well. But I am blind. I then anointed her eyes, telling her that she should see the light of the day. Her sight immediately returned, and the next day, she, with her husband, was on her way to Illinois.*[5]

It likewise proved of immense benefit to those possessed with an evil spirit, and was a therapeutic measure employed to restore such raving maniacs to their sanity:

On arriving at the pa (village) we stopped at the home of the president of the branch, but were only there a few moments, when someone shouted from across the river for me to hurry and see the sick woman. I immediately crossed on the punt, and, approaching the tent where the afflicted party lay, I saw her through the door with two strong native women trying to hold her. She was pleading with them to let her go that she might flee from the presence of the "Mormon" Elder. I could sense at once by the terrible influence, that she was possessed of evil spirits. Her husband was lying on the grass about two rods from the tent door.

It might be well to say here that the Maori men are more afraid of evil spirits than are the women. The women also are often stronger physically than the average man, being accustomed to heavy outdoor work.

I approached her husband and asked why he had sent for me. He said he had not, but that our people had made the request for me to come and administer to her. I informed him that to heal the afflicted there must be faith in the hearts of those who desired the blessing, and quoted scripture to prove it; that if the ordinance was administered without faith, the blessing would not follow, and he would ridicule the Saints and their faith.

He then told me that he believed in the Bible and knew that the scriptures were there which I had quoted. Consenting to administer the ordinance, I entered the tent and told all to leave except the afflicted woman and those holding her. I felt that the powers of darkness were very strong. It required the strength of the two women to hold her. I knelt down and offered prayer and then arose and proceeded to administer the oil. SHE GRASPED THE SPOON IN HER TEETH with great violence. I succeeded however, in GETTING THE OIL INTO HER MOUTH, and as I did so the powers of darkness weakened. After anointing her head, I confirmed the same by the laying on of hands when she suddenly wilted, and had to be held from falling on the ground, when but a few moments previous she was raving with violence. The sisters prepared her a bed, and she slept quietly for about two and a half hours. This was the first sleep she had procured for several days, except for a few moments at a time in the midst of which she would start violently and rise up in a raving condition.[6]

Some Elders in the Church had expressed opinions other than what a mighty Prophet of God had first introduced among the people earlier:

A young lady in one of our Sunday Schools informed her teacher that an Elder had rebuked her for using consecrated oil to rub her own throat with. His reason for doing so, as he said, was that she had no right to use oil in that way; it must be used only in the hands of the Priesthood.

It seems incredible that any Elder should utter such a rebuke, and we think there must be some mistake about this statement; for such a rebuke would be nothing less than bigotry. A man must be densely ignorant who would make any such remarks.[7]

However, there have been plenty of the young people in Zion who believed in these things, and continued to attach the same reverence and respect towards them as Joseph Smith had done in his day. One Mormon lad of eight years of age, Levi Lorenzo Savage by name, testified to its use in his family in the following interesting manner:

I will endeavor to relate to you how my baby sister was healed of sore eyes.

Mamma had been anointing the baby's eyes with consecrated oil. But one of the neighbors said, "You might just as well pour warm water into her eyes as to put oil on them."

Different remedies were recommended to Mamma for the baby's eyes, but the more she heard, the more faith she seemed to have, and felt in her heart and said that she knew the consecrated oil was the best. She again anointed the baby's eyes with the oil and prayed God to heal them up. Her prayer was answered, for the baby's eyes were well the next morning, and looked as though they had never been sore. And they were swollen and inflamed very badly before this.

This instance of healing has increased my faith in this ordinance of the gospel.[8]

Children in those days loved the prophets and believed that what they taught were the right things to do. The successors of Joseph Smith carried on his philosophy and doctrine in regards to the internal use of consecrated olive oil, and successive generations of little ones after him came to have faith in his teachings and great confidence in his words.

> *There is a little circumstance that happened a week or two ago to my little boy that I will relate. He will be six years old next month. He was playing in the yard and fell on a broken bottle and cut his leg. It was quite a bad cut for the time. The wound laid open and the flesh hanging out. Of course, mother-like, I was frightened. He was crying, but the first words he said to me were, "Ma, I don't want no doctor to fix my leg."*
>
> *So I said, "What do you want, Charley?" He said he wanted some oil. "What oil?" I said. Of course, I knew that he meant consecrated oil. "That will make me better." I applied the oil and in half an hour he was up running around again. I was afraid that it would start bleeding again, but it did not. It was astonishing how it healed.*
>
> *This shows that he has great faith in the oil and he will DRINK THE OIL LIKE WATER. I always use to give it to them from their infancy, and I know it does them good. This little circumstance makes me think more than ever of my boy; and how thankful we ought to feel to our Heavenly Father for our precious jewels, when we can observe the light and knowledge He bestows upon them and will continue so to do if we only keep His commandments and strive to teach our children to do the same.*[9]

When a child was injured in some way, or just unusually restless, nothing seemed to satisfy it more than a teaspoonful of olive oil, which would soothe the excited youngster down into a gentle slumber very soon:

> *Thursday, January 9, 1890. Scott is just learning to walk, consequently gets a good many falls. He got one today and he must have rammed something into his mouth when he fell. But seemed all right until evening when he began to cry and he could not be pacified for two or three hours. Emily gave him some CONSECRATED OIL INTERNALLY, and put the blessed handkerchief around his neck. He soon quieted down and went to sleep. All seemed all right ever since. He scarcely ever cries...that made us worry more than we otherwise have done.*[11]

There are many more accounts which might be offered to demonstrate the extensive use of this natural product in the Mormon way of life. However, these few illustrations should suffice for now.

Olive oil, while part of the pioneer need, was basically a necessity of secular use and religious purpose. Unlike other things of Nature which have been previously discussed in this book, this particular item was taken in faith, not in hunger.

However, the importance of olive oil is not to be underestimated in the sense of just plain nutritive value. Government research conducted by the U.S. Department of Agriculture has revealed that one cup of pure, virgin olive oil contains *AN ASTONISHING 1,945 CALORIES*! Furthermore, *IT RANKS SECOND* in high food energy content out of all of the other natural foods listed in their charts. Oily rich dairy cream came in first with 2,635 calories.[12] With such an amazing show of figures, it is easily seen why olive oil as an important food source for quick energy cannot be disputed nor argued. And the nice thing about this is that it is *COMPLETELY NATURAL*, being devoid of any kind of impurities or additives whatsoever. Certainly, the inclusion of this every morning in one's diet, with say a tablespoon or two, would be well worth the health-minded investigating.

Times have changed and so have people. Today the consumption of this vital, life-giving element into the human system is no longer practiced. Doctor's medicines and prescribed drugs have replaced what another generation considered to be the sure "remedy of God" for whatever ailed them. Now the use of consecrated olive oil is only relegated to the crown of the head, upon which the Elders of the Church place a drop when administering to the sick. Otherwise, its use in any other form is discouraged and not recommended.

At present, Joseph Smith's original use of olive oil in a most liberal manner is not too common a practice. Despite this, the injunction given by Jesus Christ will always hold true, no matter what men in any age may feel inclined to do otherwise: "*THEY THAT ARE FOOLISH TAKE NO OIL; BUT THE WISE TOOK OIL IN THEIR VESSELS*!"[13] Or, as the Savior put it another way: "Wisdom is justified of all her children."[14]

NOTES

1. Matthew 25:3 (Inspired Version).

2. I Thessalonians 4:4.

3. *Juvenile Instructor* 47:66.

4. *The Deseret Weekly* 49:127.

5. N.B. Lundwall, *Faith Like The Ancients*; Manti, 1973; p. 215.

6. *Juvenile Instructor* 24:283.

7. *Juvenile Instructor* 29:242.

8. *Ibid.*, 30:613.

9. *Woman's Exponent* 12:142. Emma J. Blunimel, Logan, Utah, February 14, 1884.

10. Early Latter-day Saints believed in the efficacy of certain articles of clothing or apparel which had been especially blessed by the Priesthood of God. One such instance involved the Prophet Joseph Smith blessing his handkerchief and giving it to Apostle Wilford Woodruff to take to a nonmember's home some distance from Commerce (Nauvoo), Illinois, where the man's children were burning up with fever and slowly dying. As it happened, though, he was fortunate enough to arrive in the nick of time, wiped their faces and brows with the sacred article of cloth entrusted into his care, and immediately the fever broke, and they began to mend from that hour forth. (See *Life of Wilford Woodruff*, p. 106)

11. *Diary of Emily Dow Partridge Young*, p. 85. Harold Lee Library, BYU, Provo.

12. *Nutritive Value of Foods*, pp. 8, 33. USDA Home and Garden Bulletin No. 72, Janaury 1971, Washing ton, D.C.

13. Matthew 25:3.

14. Luke 7:35.

CHAPTER NINE

BETTER THAN MEAT

(Fibrous Foods in L.D.S. Use)

The following items are considered by leading nutritionists to be a part of that group high in fibrous content: the legumes, corn, potatoes, and bean sprouts. The value of such articles has been lauded by doctors and medical researchers as having significant worth in eliminating certain kinds of physical problems from the system of man, which the "soft type" of foods has caused. Reliable authorities have determined that such conditions as hiatal hernia, appendicitis, and cancer of the colon were virtually non-existent in the pioneer days. And this was due to the amount of roughage in the food of those days, which these people consumed. It is actually thought by many medical experts that such fibrous material within the system actually cleanses the body in a way so as to remove toxic poisons from the system. A rough comparison would be to the harsh abrasives used in cleaning and scouring. Though the action is somewhat different, yet the principle is the same—roughage gets rid of the improper matter!

The Legumes

Perhaps nothing is better suited for the human system than these. Rich in protein and important as a major source for body energy, they could be rightfully classified as "better than meat" for what they have to offer. Leah D. Widstoe commented about their use in this way:

> *The legumes—peas, beans, lentils —are also valuable protein foods. They are the richest source of vegetable protein, containing about 25% protein; and while not classed as a "complete protein" as are eggs, milk, or meat, yet they are very valuable in the normal diet. The soy bean is an exception, inasmuch as it contains some of the constituents of a complete protein, and it forms an alkaline reaction in digestion, whereas most other proteins are decidedly acid-formers. The soy bean has formed the basis of the protein requirement of the Chinese*

people for many millenniums.

The best nourishment results when the proteins of different foods are taken in combination; therefore, the legumes are valuable for complete nutrition. If properly cooked, THEY MAY OFTEN TAKE THE PLACE OF MEAT—especially when milk and eggs form part of the diet. Besides being a source of protein, legumes are rich in vitamins and minerals—especially the precious vitamin B complex.

There are many varieties of edible dried legumes, such as navy, kidney, pink, red, black eye, yellow eye, lima and soy beans; Scotch peas, split peas, cow peas, black peas, and lentils. They are generally inexpensive, and under proper conditions will keep almost indefinitely. Indeed, THEY ARE ONE OF THE BEST FOODS TO STORE AND KEEP IN RESERVE FOR A TIME OF WANT![1]

Many Latter-day Saints who go to great efforts to secure for themselves an adequate food storage in times of famine could do well to pay heed to the wise counsel offered by Sister Widstoe. So many families nowadays purchase large quantities of dehydrated foods in various forms. Whether packaged or canned, these products have been prepared under nitrogen, which renders them into a state where they won't spoil or deteriorate. This may be fine for the consumer as a handy convenience to insure a long shelf-life, but it is not a very wise measure to incorporate into one's own life and system upon consumption. For the nitrogen contained in the foodstuffs can lead to serious health problems later on, and consequential illness if one is not careful about their use.

The *natural* thing to do would be as Sister Widstoe has so soundly suggested, and that is to lay up a store and reserve of *LEGUMES* in preference to dehydrated foods. Early Latter-day Saints, who could travel with very little, relied heavily upon such items for continued sustenance and lasting strength. An example, for instance, is the type of fare which the Danish converts migrating to Utah in the early 1860s had to subsist upon while crossing the ocean: "Many emigrants were loaded on the ship *Monarch of the Sea* which left April 28, 1864. The Church had bought our provisions—hardtack, pork, PEAS, and a little flour, sugar, coffee, and a few other things."[2] And when the Saints were crossing the plains in '47, various kinds of dried beans were sometimes the only food they ever saw for periods at a time:

President Young gave notice that those who wanted to send to St. Louis had better make out their bills and send them in soon; there was a feeling of distrust among the Saints about honest dealing; and if any man said we dealt dishonestly, he lied and he knew he lied before God. "For two years, while the Twelve have been building," said the President, "they have paid, when they borrowed, as they have agreed to. A man apostatized and returned to Nauvoo and said Elder Kimball had stolen all his BEANS. Elder Heber C. Kimball put TWO BUSHELS OF BEANS in his wagon for him to haul and afterwards went and distributed them to the poor, and the man apostatized."[3]

Lentils were also an important item of food with which their daily hunger seemed to be adequately sustained:

Mrs. Orson Hyde invited our family to breakfast one morning out of politeness as she knew we had no way of getting any; people owing Dr. Williams in promises that did not feed us. They did not realize when they were eating, we were hungry and rightly owned some of their store. Sister Vilate Kimball, I saw every day, picking greens and came to see how much provisions I had. I had a pint of ground barley I showed her. She said Brother Kimball had given her a nice sack of lentils to divide with those who were really needy. She sent 3 quarts to me. I sent half to the Farm as Mother Williams was cooking for the men. I indulged in cooking some for myself and the children. It was good.[4]

Thus we are able to see that in times of dire hardship, such as the early Mormon pioneers faced, the legumes of beans, peas, and lentils formed a very necessary part of their diets. And yet, from all indications, it seems that their general health was apparently quite good, for they did not suffer from any types of improper nourishment while eating these sustaining elements of food. This, together with various kinds of whole grain products (such as wheat bread, oatmeal, and boiled barley in place of coffee) provided them with ample nutrition of a selected quality.

For those of us, then, who are anticipating some program of future food storage, or adding to our present supply, it would be well to investigate the possibility of such worthy additions in our own homes. After all, the distinct advantage to these acquisitions over commercial products of dehydrated value is simply that *THEY ARE NATURAL* to begin with at the time of purchase, and *REMAIN NATURAL AT THE TIME OF STORAGE*!

A combination of grains and legumes has a secondary value, also:

> *People who live in Mexico, India, or the Middle East have long known the value of combining grains and legumes. For centuries they have thrived on rice, wheat, corn and all types of beans, peas and lentils. Each culture has developed its own distinctive combination of herbs and spices to flavor native vegetables, meat dishes and the ubiquitous grain-legume pairing.*
>
> *In this country we have become very excited in the last few years about the concept of complementary proteins—the idea that those very grains, when combined with those self-same beans, peas and lentils, can produce a protein of quality equal to that of old ground round and more expensive T-bones and roasts. What's the reason behind this amazing feat performed by these humble plant products? Complementary amino acids, the building blocks of protein. For example, grains, nuts and seeds are all deficient in iso-leucine and lysine, while legumes contain an abundance of these two amino acids—which are plentiful in grains, nuts and seeds. Therefore, eating a grain such as rice or wheat in the same meal with beans, peas, or lentils, seasoned with sesame seeds, adds up to a very high-quality protein meal—comparable to meat or eggs.*
>
> *In adition to providing balanced protein, such a meal can be exciting to the eye and palate,and may be closer to the ideal diet for all the world's people than the typical American meat-centered diet with its high energy cost for raising, refining and processing foods. When it relies on whole grains, such a diet also provides fiber or roughage, now shown to be essential for a healthy digestive tract. Cutting down on our consumption of meats and saturated fats would help keep our hearts healthy.*[5]

Similar views have been sustained by leading Church authorities of the past. In the *Latter-day Saints' Millennial Star* of 1931, advice was offered by the Prophet, President Heber J. Grant, that "meat should be eaten sparingly." Also strong recommendations for a "balanced diet," which would include "1/6 protein, 1/6 fat, and 2/3's carbohydrates" was specifically urged. Furthermore, it was emphasized in the article that the protein portion should be "*DIVIDED BETWEEN ANIMAL AND VEGETABLE PROTEIN,*" stressing "*PEAS, BEANS, LENTILS...*" as some of the items for the second kind of protein. And after the carbohydrate allotment of two-thirds, *WHOLE-GRAIN* cereals was included in a list of several other items, all enclosed in parenthesis.[6]

Yet despite this evidence and proof, many will find old habits hard to break. The way in which most are presently accustomed to eating, unfortunately, will remain the same. However, for those whose will is stronger to change than others, once convinced of the truth, the following facts are offered from the scriptures for careful consideration.

FACT: When Daniel and his three friends were offered the heavy meat and fine bread diet of the Babylonians, they instead chose a diet consisting of nothing more than plain simple legumes and some kind of uncooked grain, with ordinary water as their drink. The full account is to be found in Daniel 1:1-20. "Pulse," as it is mentioned in the Bible, means "peas, beans, and the seeds that grow in pods. Probably the term denotes uncooked grain of any kind, as barley, wheat, millet, vetches, etc."[7]

Or, as another Bible scholar proffered: "The word means simply 'seeds'...as peas, and other *LEGUMINOUS VEGETABLES. IT WAS SIMPLY A PLAIN VEGETABLE DIET THAT DANIEL AND HIS FRIENDS REQUESTED*!"[8]

FACT: That after Daniel told Melzar, in whose custody they were, to try them this way for ten days and then let the king decide between them and the rest who had been fed the Babylonian way, Nebuchanezar found the four young Israelites *TEN TIMES BETTER* than all the rest in his realm.[9] They *EXCEEDED* everyone else in wisdom, knowledge and understanding, not to mention their fair complexions and good countenances.

FACT: King David, the shepherd boy, while in his youth, ate of these things, too.

> *And it came to pass, when David was come to Mahanaim, that Shobi the son of Nahash of Rabbah of the children of Ammon, and Machir, the son of Ammiel of Lo-debar, and Barzillai the Gileadite of Rogelim,*
>
> *Brought beds, and basins and earthen vessels, and wheat, and barley, and flour, and PARCHED CORN AND BEANS, AND LENTILES, AND PARCHED PULSE,*
>
> *And honey, and butter, and sheep, and cheese of kine, for David, and for the people that were with him, TO EAT; for they said, The people is hungry, and weary, and thirsty, in the wilderness.*[10]

The Biblical commentator who expresses himself upon this issue says, in part, that "...parched peas are a favorite diet in the East. Pulse or peas of many kinds are, and always were, cultivated in Palestine."[11]

FACT: That from such a diet as this, young David was the epitome of good, sound health *WHICH SHOULD BE IN EVERYONE OF GOD'S CHILDREN UPON THE EARTH*! No acne or pimpled face in this one, nor blanched expression of outward looks either, which is so common among our youth today, including many Mormon teenagers:

> *Now he (David) was RUDDY, and withal of A BEAUTIFUL COUNTENANCE, and GOODLY TO LOOK TO!*[12]

And together with what information we have available concerning the Prophet Joseph Smith's great physical stamina and tremendous vigor, we can safely say that *THESE THREE MEN OF GOD*—Daniel, David, and Joseph Smith—*ATE IN SUCH A WAY AS TO PROMOTE GOOD HEALTH WITHIN THEIR SYSTEMS IN ORDER TO ENJOY THE SPECIAL BLESSINGS OF GOD UPON THEM, IN A SPIRITUAL WAY!*

The use of the legumes and whole-grain products in modern L.D.S. diet is not as extensive as it once was among the early Saints. Too many of us have gone the way the majority of Judah did in the days of Daniel, when they ate the food of Babylon instead of the nourishing things which God expected His Children, Israel, to consume. Now, this is not the opinion of the author, but merely an echo of a similar sentiment expressed by a former pioneer of great fame. Joel Johnson, who authored the familiar "High On The Mountain Top," had this to say about modern-day Israel becoming so much like the world in so many different ways:

> *January 21, 1873 Went down to St. George to see the President and...attend a two day meeting to be held on the following Saturday and Sunday in the St. George Tabernacle...I was truly thankful to see the beginning made to induce the saints to obey the first commandment given to the Church that was to "come out of Babylon, Oh my people, be ye seperate; touch not, taste not, hear not of her unclean things." THIS COMMANDMENT THE CHURCH AS A PEOPLE HAVE NEVER KEPT! For that cause we have been robbed and driven, from place to place and still the spirit of the king is after us; WE HAVE CONSTANTLY SOUGHT AFTER THE UNCLEAN THINGS OF THE GENTILES OF BABYLON, SUCH AS THEIR BACON AND ALL THE ROUND OF THEIR CANDY AND BOTTLED FRUITS*

AND PROVISIONS, with their clothing, fashions, manners, customs and many of their practices while the Lord hath said that those things were unclean and not good for man and that the beauty of our appearance should be the workmanship of our own fingers, while we continue to follow after Babylon the spirit of Babylon will follow us and our children and we cannot help ourselves. I have refused to use their unclean things and to follow their fashions for the last forty years and have always preached against it and feel thankful that the first step is taken to bring the saints out of Babylon...[13]

As previously stated in the opening pages of this book, President George Q. Cannon, a member of the First Presidency, emphatically stated "that if we wish to raise a healthy, noble looking, intellectual and perfect race of men and women *WE MUST FEED OUR CHILDREN PROPERLY!*"[14]

With both of these dynamic testimonies before us, how can we refuse to do otherwise? How can we continue in the dark of our present ignorance, with the light before us? The scriptures say, "light cleaveth to light, and truth to truth." If we are of the light, and love the light of revealed knowledge and proper wisdom, will we not discontinue our current methods of careless eating in lieu of something better? In short, the fact is simply this: If we *TRULY ARE* what we profess to be—the people of God—then we will adjust our diets to include those things which Daniel and David and Joseph Smith ate, to guarantee us good health for this life and a better kingdom in the world to come through our faithful obedience and strict adherance to His laws of sound nutrition and proper eating.

Corn was also another natural food product which the Latter-day Saints enjoyed. Sometimes it was the only thing they had to eat.

After we left Far West, we were left alone for awhile. The mob worried to know where my father was. One day a deputation of men came to our place and generously gave father three days to get away, which pleased us very much for we certainly had no desire to stay. Father was an expert in everything he tried to do, and he rigged up a foot lathe and soon had two hubs turned out. It didn't take us long to build a cart, and soon we were traveling off with the cart box filled with CORN. The snow was deep enough to take me to the middle of the thigh, and I was bare footed, and in my shirt tail. Mother had made me a tow shirt in Kirtland, and the shirt still stuck to me, or rather, I still stuck to the shirt. We had old Tom hitched to the cart, and father drove the horse and carried the rifle on his shoulder. Mother followed the cart carrying my little brother, Francis Marion, in her arms. I tried to follow in her tracks. We finally stopped to rest and get something to eat; but mother said she could not stand it much longer. She cried...and father said, "Cheer up, Clarissa, for I prophesy in the name of the Lord Jesus Christ—you shall have a pair of shoes delivered to you before long, in a remarkable manner!"

After we had made our fire and eaten of our ROASTED CORN ON THE COB, mother reached down on the side to get her old shoes, and held up a new pair! Father answered, "Clarissa, did I not tell you that God would provide you a pair in a remarkable manner?" We continued on until dark when we found a good sized log to build our bed by. Our cart was filled with EARS OF CORN, so we could not make our bed in it. We made a bed of leaves and put a quilt on top of them, then we covered ourselves with what loose garments we could spare—we were not over-supplied with clothing in those days. Father had what was called in those days a coat; I had my shirt; and mother had one dress made of the same material as my shirt. She had made them in Kirtland, and since that time hadn't had the opportunity to spin or weave because the mob would not give us time to get anything together. We even had to leave our flax after we had raised it! Father cut down a basswood tree for Tom to graze on during the night.

We gathered elmbark to eat with our CORN ON THE COB—elmbark and buds helped us get along until we came to the Mississippi River. There we camped for the night because we didn't know how to cross the river. Oh! what a cold night that was! Tom had some buds and limbs to browse on; and we still had some corn left. We found some herbs growing on strings which we discovered to be wild potatoes—they were good roasted, but I was glad to eat what I could find raw. We also had elmbark which was a luxury with CORN.[15]

However, in modern times, something so simple as corn has ceased to be a precious commodity and rather instead has become an extra item to be pushed aside with an upturned nose, or discarded at random.

Richard Holley, an 11th-grade student at Springville High School, recently informed the author that while working in the lunch room many trays came back with food still left on them, among which was a numerous amount of untouched creamed corn, as the particular vegetable for that day's menu. He said this was a typical thing to see and stated that "some trays were still full when they returned. You wouldn't believe the waste," he concluded in disgust.[16]

Now such a practice is quite common in the United States today, with hundreds of thousands of American school children. A further example of such careless waste may be seen in an elementary school located in Camarillo, California:

> *An elementary school principal in this agricultural community became distressed by watching pupils toss most or part of their lunches into the garbage can.*
>
> *To dramatize the waste, principal Jerry Moyniham gathered the pupils and teachers of Pleasant Valley school around a picnic table during a recent lunch hour. He dumped the contents of the nearest trash can onto the table.*
>
> *Among other items, out rolled large, unpeeled oranges, shiny red apples with not a bite missing and an assortment of neatly wrapped sandwiches.*
>
> *Sixth grader Arlene Medina prepared the official inventory:*
>
> *There were 41 sandwiches, two burritos, two cartons of milk, two whole pieces of chicken, three bags of potato chips, 19 apples, 13 oranges, one piece of cake, a half can of chocolate pudding, four carrot pieces, a piece of Mexican bread, two small boxes of raisins, 19 pieces of candy and 14 cookies.*[17]

Such flagrant abuse with the bounties of Nature's harvest is not just relegated to the Gentile populations alone. In the predominantly Mormon state of Utah, this repeated occurrence happens too frequently, and, sadly enough, it involves large scores of LDS children besides.

> *One of the favorite sayings of school teacher, Clay Petersen's mother when he was growing up, was "Waste not, want not."*
>
> *"I'm afraid Americans will be wanting a lot before long if they continue to waste food the way they are wasting it now,"*

he says.

"There is enough waste among our school children alone to feed Europe's and Asia's starving children," says Petersen.

Petersen is a sixth grade teacher at John C. Fremont Elementary School, 4249 S. 1425 West (Salt Lake City). He has carefully measured and weighed the food wasted at his school on three different occasions.

"If every school were the same as ours, and I know a lot are even worse, then UTAH'S SCHOOLS would WASTE MORE THAN 14 TONS OF FOOD AND ABOUT 2,500 GALLONS OF MILK EVERY DAY!

"Multiply that by 50 states—most of them alot bigger than Utah, too—and you will find the amount of food wasted in our school systems extraordinary," says Petersen.

Recently Petersen's students were on kitchen detail at their school. At the end of each lunch period they weighed the amount of food thrown away (which did not include paper or non-food items) and also measured the milk thrown away.

"We were very careful to measure just food waste. We measured the amount of milk wasted by having each child pour the remaining contents of his or her milk container into a special pail," Petersen explained.

On Monday, 512 students bought school lunches and ate them in the school cafeteria. We had sloppy Joe hamburgers, potato chips, carrots, oatmeal cookies and half an apple in addition to milk that day," said Petersen.

Students wasted a total of 58.5 pounds of food and threw away 7.3 gallons of milk.

The other day's waste was recorded as follows:

Tuesday: 86.75 pounds of food, 8.25 gallons of milk; Wednesday: 88 pounds of food and 8.3 gallons of milk; Thursday: 89 pounds of food and 9.66 gallons of milk; and Friday: 110 pounds of food and 3.6 gallons of milk.

The total waste for the week, Petersen's students found, was 431 pounds of food and 37.25 gallons of milk. Total number of persons eating in the lunchroom during the week, including some adults and a few kindergarten students, was 2,790.

Petersen extrapolated his figures to Utah, using the figure 180,000 as the number of students in the state participating in the school lunch program.

"I believe the figures are conservative. Fremont School is just an average school as far as income is concerned. I would suspect the more affluent neighborhoods in the state would contribute even more waste," said Petersen.

Petersen grew up on a farm near Moab in San Juan County. His father died when he was young and his mother raised him and his four brothers.

"We didn't have much to eat in those days and we tried to make the most of everything," said Petersen.

"WE AMERICANS WASTE EVERYTHING! Food is one of the most vital commodities wasted."[18]

Quite obviously, corn was in there somewhere, too.

But it just does not end here with youth. Unfortunately, it carries over into the adult group likewise. When the author worked in the restaurant business several years ago, he was dinner chef for a brief period of time at the Riverside Country Club in Provo, Utah. It was the holiday season of Thanksgiving and Christmas, and many party and banquet reservations had been made well in advance. While catering to a women's church auxiliary organization, common in the valley, he noticed how so many of the ladies pushed the quarter cob of corn aside on their plates, or utterly refused to touch it altogether. Many precious ears of a vital substance went into the garbage disposal that day, including good portions of remaining petite filet mignons as well, which had been served as the main luncheon course for that gathering.

This section was not prepared to discuss the mineral and vitamin content of corn, but rather to show the absolute waste of which so many people, including a large number of Mormon families, are thoroughly guilty of commiting. While it may seem to some as a personal tirade against others, yet this is not the purpose for citing the evidence just given. Rather it is for the sole objective of instilling within the hearts and minds of everyone concerned with such neglectful habits, a desire to conserve rather than waste.

The big thing these days seems to be conservation. The printed media, as well as screen, broadcasts messages of timely importance upon this very subject, at regular intervals. One well-known actor, in fact, is constantly seen on Utah Power & Light advertisements stressing the careful use of electricity. "Use what you need, but *NEED* what you use," he charms in a methodical way.

Such, then, ought to be our slogan too, in regards to food—any kind of food—and its daily consumption by all of us. We should "use what we need, but *NEED* what we use." Also, an attitude of greater reverence and respect is needed for Him whose plant creations we waste so abundantly. Plus, a more grateful heart for the food we eat is wanting in everyone. Our attitude and disposition towards these things should be precisely what Father Smith's was, in relation to a lowly ear of corn once:

> *This summer Brother Joseph came home, and we went up to his place to see him. As I glanced on his table and beheld a beautiful boiled corn on the cob, I thought, "Oh, what a grand sight!" The corn seemed to be of the King Phillip variety of yellow flint. Brother Joseph asked his father to return thanks on the food, and Father Smith took up an ear of corn in his right hand holding it between his thumb and forefinger, and said, "Oh, God, the Eternal Father, we thank thee for this corn, and pray in the name of Jesus Christ to bless it to the strengthening of our bodies, and the strengthening of our stomachs till Thou can provide something better; which we ask of Thee in the name of Jesus Christ, Amen." Tears were streaming down his cheeks, and I thought it a repast of the most excellent type.*[19]

In ancient times corn was ground the old-fashioned way, by cattle yoked to stone mills and as they walked in a circle, the stone would slowly turn, thereby grinding whatever was put into it. Occasionally, some would spill over the side and fall into the dirt. Under ordinary circumstances it would go to waste. But God made a special provision, whereby not even a kernel would be lost. He instructed the Hebrew children: "Thou shalt not muzzle the ox when he treadeth out the corn."[20] By employing this measure, nothing was lost, for the animal would eat that which had fallen upon the ground as it continued in its tiring walk around the circle. Therefore, if *GOD DOES NOT SANCTION WASTE*, how can we tolerate it amongst ourselves so easily as we do?

Potatoes

"It is only a few hundred years since the potato was discovered, and what a blessing it has proven to man!"[21] So said Apostle George Q. Cannon. The potato was as important as the pioneers themselves, and finds a proper place in history alongside those first emigrants to enter the valley in '47:

> *George A. Smith was six weeks without bread, though he had twenty-five pounds of flour locked up in his trunk unknown to others. This reserve of flour he distributed by cupfuls to the sick of the company, several of whom owed the preservation of their lives to this action.*
>
> *He devoted great attention to the sick and the poor. When in Winter Quarters, Iowa, the people suffered greatly from disease, through lack of vegetable diet. He urged the cultivation of the potato as a remedy, and under his advice the small quantity of seed that could be obtained was planted, the yield being marvelously heavy. He was familiarly called "the potato Saint," and on his arrival in the Great Salt Lake valley he planted the first potatoes put into Utah soil.*[22]

In many ways the potato was a life-saver. Not necessarily would the Saints have to eat it, in order for it to prove beneficial in this regard:

> *They left Liverpool on April 20, 1863, on the ship John J. Boyd in company with 755 Saints under the direction of William Duff. They were five weeks on the water. Mary was seven years old and told the following incident: One day a whale came up to the vessel and raised its head up, leaning against the boat. The Captain ordered all the people to go to the opposite side of of the ship so it wouldn't tip over, then ordered some of the men to bring buckets of potatoes, which they poured into the whale's mouth until finally it slid back into the water and went away.*[23]

Potato was regarded in the same manner as grain, and Latter-day Saints considered them both of equal importance. As Wilford Woodruff observed, "When we came here our position demanded that the very first thing we did was to plant our potatoes and sow our wheat, or we had starvation before us." Food supplies may have been scarce at times, but it seems there was always plenty of potatoes on hand.[25]

The pioneers had different methods of fixing spuds. One old-timer fondly recalled: "We had many meals of roasted potatoes in the ashes, salt and water."[26] Some of the Mormon Battalion boys enjoyed a tasty repast of "boiled rawhide soup, with frozen potatoes, and laced by an addition of ripe rosebuds encased in ice."[27] The author himself has found that left-over mashed potatoes may be whipped up in the blender with a little milk added to thin the consistency somewhat, then heated and served later on as homemade potato soup, with a few spices thrown in for good seasoning measure. And the *Millennial Star*, a Mormon publication, suggests another type of "potato soup with the peelings left in" for better nutrition.[28]

Meat and potatoes has always been one of the tasty dishes which man has been very fond of. The Latter-day Saints incorporated this as part of their diet, too. Potatoes found themselves accompanying an interesting variety of meat dishes down through Mormon history. These have ranged all the way from the bizarre—Joseph Smith and his associates being served what the mobocrats termed as "Mormon roast" and potatoes, which was nothing more than the cooked flesh of a deceased colored man, given them while incarcerated in Liberty Jail[29]—to the downright ludicrous:

> *...when I came (August 20, 1865), my mother being a frail and delicate woman, rather than have me follow the other two, concurred the idea of letting the Indian women diggers and Pleades take me and nurse me along with the balance of the papooses and did I thrive, well did I? I now weigh nigh unto 225 lbs., and one of the childish recollections of mine was when one of those squaws would sling me on her back with another papoose and strike out in the sandflats and proceed to catch their dinner by using a long iron rod with a hook on one end and reach down the rat holes around the mesquite bushes and hook the ground squirrels and bull lizards and pull them out and throw them in the fire, kicking and squealing, guts, feathers and all, and when roasted to their liking, take them out with some wild potatoes, and give each of us papooses one to gnaw on, be it squirrel or bull lizard. And believe me, if I didn't get my part of the nurse from the breast of one of these squaws or my part of the roasted squirrel or bull lizard and potatoes, war was immediately declared between the whites and the Indians, and as I seem to remember, I always got my share or more.* [30]

Elder Jonathan Dunham recorded in his journal of 1843, while upon a special mission to the Indian tribes along the western Missouri, that "in the morning we got a few potatoes and boiled them. I killed two grey squirrels and the squaw burned off the hair, and boiled them."[31] However, it seems apparent that these Indians were a bit more particular about how they cleaned the animal than were the root-diggers of the Utah Territory.

Meat and potatoes served as prison food for those in jail. Orin Porter Rockwell fared a little better than what his friends had done in Liberty. While being held in a Missouri dungeon, he fished for pukes from the nearby river, to go along with his regular staple of bread and potatoes.[32]

William C. Staines, while residing among the Ponca nation one winter, found the meat and potatoes a pleasurable change from immediate starvation. The spuds he didn't mind, but the meat—well, that was something else and took a little more getting use to: "They think skunk meat very fine food. I have been called up at midnight to go to a skunk feast. When dressed and cooked properly the meat is good; if not cooked properly it is very strong, so much so that one can taste it the next day after eating it." Apparently, this is one meal that would always "stay with a person."

Heber McBride, another old duffer of years gone by, remembered a dinner of roast badger and potatoes he and his companion had one winter.[43]

Potatoes, in combination with several other simple food items of natural source, can be a major factor in good health and reduce the immediate possibilities of sickness or disease. Though the Mormon pioneers had this and a few dairy products with the natural greens which they dug from the nearby hills, yet their health seemed to maintain a consistency proportionately higher than our level of standard currently is.

Similar conditions have been experienced today by others in isolated conditions, such as what the early settlers to this state first were:

> *In 1932, nearly 84 percent of the residents of the island of Tristan da Cunha in the South Atlantic were free of tooth decay. In less than thirty years, the level of decay has risen sharply to that usually encountered in sophisticated societies, apparently in direct relation to the rise in imported food, particularly flour and sugar.*
>
> *Last month the island was evacuated because of a*

volcanic eruption, ending the thirty-year study of the teeth of the islanders. They have been resettled in the village of Merttham in Surrey and their bad teeth are being cared for free by dentists of the British National Health Service.

Though the island was far from a paradise in any normal sense, the conditions existing there when the first dental survey was made in 1932 by officers of the British Battleship Carlisle were considered to be ideal for the growth and preservation of healthy teeth.

The islanders were entirely dependent for food on their own resources. Fish were abundant. Scanty pastures supported cattle, sheep, geese and hens. Eggs were collected from seabirds. A few cabbages, onions and turnips were grown. But THE STAPLE CROP WAS POTATOES!

Having neither currency nor the means to barter with the outside world, the inhabitants were confined to a home grown diet of eggs, milk, fish, meat AND POTATOES...

But since then the dental state of the islanders has steadily deteriorated in the direct relation to the rise in the amount of imported food.[35]

It is an interesting thing to observe that almost the same identical things have happened with the Latter-day Saints. When they first came into the valley, they lived on potatoes, wheat, simple greens, milk, eggs and occasional cheese. But as the taste for "the unclean things of the Gentiles in Babylon, such as their bacon, candy, and bottled fruits and provisions" began to increase more among the Mormon people (according to previous testimony of Joel Johnson), a similar increase in their dental problems and health care was to be noticed, likewise. More doctors, advertisements in the local paper and dentists' shingles hung out on Main Street became quite evident in the years to follow. Thus, our present condition of poor health and nutrition is due, in part, to the inadequate diet of our ancestors.

A strict diet of potatoes or any kind of starchy food is not good. Declared Elder George Q. Cannon: "A people who, for instance, are fed on potatoes alone do not have the stamina that they would have if they had a greater variety of food." Furthermore, he added, "Such a people could...be kept subjected more easily to thralldom than a nation which is better fed."[36]

Now, the dictionary defines "thralldom" as "a state of moral or mental slavery or bondage." It also says that this can be "one bound as by habit; a slave."[37] Both definitions are now archaic and no longer in use in the English language. However, it does point up a very interesting fact in regards to our present generation of young people.

Considering that the diet of the normal teenager today is mostly starch (french-fried potatoes, hamburger and hotdog buns, etc.) and very little protein (some meat, but usually the wrong kind, such as what could easily be purchased from any drive-in or take-out stand), is it any wonder that the present generation of American youth are subjected to the poor habits of lousy nutrition, and veritable slaves to the commercial system which caters such garbage for convenience sake? Big busines food advertisements have replaced the common-sense wisdom that whispered so carefully to our forefathers many decades ago. And it would seem, from all indications, that the children of modern day Israel are a part of this "thralldom" too.

The plain fact is *WE DO NOT EAT RIGHT*, and it's about time we faced up to the issues, instead of ducking them every time our stomach says "feed me!" We need to return to a sound diet of logical nutrition in order to bring about a better state of health than what we have previously, heretofore, seemingly "enjoyed."

This does not necessarily need to involve a mad rush for the local health food store in order to stock up on the "right" kind of stuff. True, they have those things which will greatly aid us in the pursuit of what we are after. But of a greater truth still, the local supermarket can yet yield an abundance of good things to eat, if we are careful in our selections and smart in our shopping. For many on limited incomes or with large families this would be the only recourse to follow. By including such things as more vegetables and fresh fruits from the produce section, and avoiding the canned foods department as much as possible, some relief may be obtained of beneficial value later on.

And then, too, the manner in which such items of Nature are prepared has a lot to do with what our bodies obtain in the way of vitamins and minerals.

Sister Leah D. Widstoe, a wise homemaker in her own time, suggested that vegetables should not be overcooked; leafy parts, such as celery, to be used in soups or salads and never discarded; and, finally, *POTATOES* to be cooked or baked *WITH THEIR SKINS OR JACKETS LEFT ON*! For directly beneath the epidermis lies the TOTAL value of its entire substance!

Bean Sprouts

Another food of natural origin is bean sprouts. Unknown to most Latter-day Saints until the early part of the twentieth century, this important item has assumed its proper role among the eating habits of the wise in Zion. Sister Leah D. Widstoe says that they are "an excellent and tasty vegetable." Also, "they are cheap and a valuable source of vitamin C."[38] In fact, she describes them thusly:

> *A vegetable that will grow in any climate, rivals meat in nutritive value, matures in three to five days, may be planted any day in the year, requires neither soil nor sunshine, rivals tomatoes in vitamin C, has no waste (in preparation), can be cooked with as little fuel and as quickly as a pork chop.*
>
> *When the sprout of the bean is about an inch or two long, much of the bean still remains. Both the bean and the sprout should be eaten.*
>
> *During sprouting, vitamin C is formed by the bean and the niacin and riboflavin (Vitamin B) increase. Sprouted beans are not likely to produce intestinal gases and thus differ from navy beans cooked in the usual way. They are also a good source of calcium.*
>
> *The great value of bean proteins has long been known. This protein must be heated to convert it to the best form. Sprouting seems to replace heating.*[39]

Several varieties of beans may be used in sprouting, among which are soy beans and mung beans. The latter seems to be the best under ideal conditions. However, alfalfa seeds also do nicely, and when used in place of lettuce on a sandwich, adds a zest and flavor to be discovered only by eating one prepared in this manner. Unlike lettuce which clings to the inside of the intestines and is hard to digest, sprouts are easily assimilated with a minimal amount of chewing involved.

To prepare sprouted beans, Sister Widstoe furnishes us with some suggestions as to the correct method and procedure, which, if carefully followed, will yield satisfying results for those who attempt it:

> *Intelligence and care must be used or the beans will mold instead of sprout.*

Whether a pound or a ton of beans are to be sprouted, two items will be needed:

1. Soy beans that will grow very rapidly. Limited tests have shown that the common field varieties, Cayuga, Seneca, and Ontario grown in New York State, will sprout well if they are of good seed quality.

2. A can of chlorinated lime, which the chemist calls calcium hydrochlorite and the housewife uses for purifying drinking water. A little of this helps to prevent mold growth, although beans can be sprouted successfully without it.

Finally, one needs a container for the sprouting beans. This should have a wide mouth for getting the beans in and out with a hole or screen in the bottom to drain off water. The producer of a pound of sprouted beans will select a flower pot, a bottle, fruit jar or bag. One who wishes to feed a hundred will use a clean, 20 gallon galvanized can with an open top and a hole cut in the bottom. The author found a churn made of earthenware to be an excellent "sprouter."

Here is the step by step process:

1. SORT BEANS, removing broken pieces and other seeds.

2. WASH BEANS.

3. SOAK BEANS OVERNIGHT in lukewarm water to cover. To one pound beans use 3 pints water and add a pinch of chlorinated lime. For 20 pounds of beans use 30 quarts of water and add 3 teaspoons chlorinated lime mixed to a paste with a little water.

4. DRAIN BEANS next morning, and pour into sprouting vessel big enough to let them swell four to six times. If a clean flower pot is used, put a piece of wire netting or cloth across the hole in the bottom. For a fruit jar, cover the opening with a zinc top punched full of holes or wire screen or cloth.

5. KEEP BEANS DARK AND MOIST. Cover the beans in the flower pot with a damp cloth. This may then be covered with a piece of damp cardboard to exclude light. If the beans are placed in a wet cloth bag, they should be suspended in a dark, damp place. If the beans are not dark, they will turn a yellowish-green.

6. WATER SEVERAL TIMES DAILY. The bottom of the flower pot or jar should be raised or tippled slightly so that all water drains out after each watering, and the beans will have air. The watering should be thorough to flush off bacterial growth. Each evening it is wise to add a pinch of chlorinated lime to the sprinkling water. Twenty pounds of beans may be sprouted in this way. For watering, a spray nozzle on the garden hose may be used. At the last wetting each night, the chlorinated lime, made into a paste, should be mixed in the water that is used for sprinkling. After the second day, the sprouting process makes the large quantity of beans warm and they should be sprinkled with cool water. For additional cooling, a cylinder of wire netting can be placed in the center of the can. During the last two days a chunk of ice can be placed on the beans.

The beans are ready to eat from the third to fifth day but in summer only two days may be needed for sprouting.

Sprouting beans should be kept refrigerated like fresh meat. For longer keeping, they may be blanched for two or three minutes, and then either frozen or canned.[40]

It may here be observed, that while Mrs. Widstoe's methods are practical, yet today there is available from large department or mercantile stores "bean sprouting kits," which include the necessary items and instructions as well. This is due, in part, to the popularity which sprouting has acquired over the years since her time.

Having reached the end of our work, it is now best to close with a short summary of all the information obtained thus far.

To begin with, only "natural foods" have been treated in this book. That is, those products derived more immediately from Nature herself. Other items, such as milk, for instance, have also been classified with the rest, simply because it too comes from Nature, only in an indirect way. It is the end result of the alfalfa and lucerne which old "Bossy" assimilates into her system and then is somehow mysteriously converted into the white substance we know after wards as "milk." In this sense, then, can it be properly filed with the rest of the foods dealt with here.

When God created man, it was His intention that he should live close to the earth which had been formed. For this reason did God put man "into the Garden of Eden, to dress it, and to keep it."[41] The science of horticulture *WAS THE VERY FIRST SCIENCE* which God taught to man. The art of growing fruits, vegetables, flowers and ornamental plants was introduced to Adam, and from the Almighty he learned how to plant seed and reap the benefits thereby. For this reason did God say to man: "Behold, I have given you every herb-bearing seed, which is upon the face of all the earth; and every tree in the which shall be the fruit of a tree, yielding seed; *TO YOU IT SHALL BE FOR MEAT.*"[42] In other words, He intended for these natural foods *TO BE BETTER THAN MEAT* for the system of man. As long as man was in obedience to these laws and natural surroundings he was able to enjoy direct communication with God upon a face-to-face basis. It was only through transgression that he lost this privilege afterwards.

From the time when the first sin was committed by Adam and Eve until now, an *UN*natural state of things has been the result. Man became blood-thirsty as a result of the curse placed upon him by His maker. A carnal disposition and an appetite for flesh replaced the more natural instincts of taste for plant life. In other words, his craving went from raw fruits and vegetables and nuts, to that of juicy, red meat. And when this happened, his open connection between Earth and Heaven became broken at last. From then on, he would have to struggle in darkness to find the spiritual light he had once enjoyed.

Now meat has its place in our diet because of the Fall. We have been told to use it "sparingly" and only in times of great famine or want. To be strictly vegetarian is not a good thing either, though it may be of tremendous help to the physical system of man. Yet for his spirit it is not such a good thing, for it allows the Evil One to do all sorts of mischief with a person's faith.

The best evidence which can be presented to show that God expects some meat in our diet because of our present fallen condition is best exemplified in the offerings of Cain and Abel. Abel, who was "a keeper of sheep" offered up an animal sacrifice—the firstlings of his flock—unto God, *"AND THE LORD HAD RESPECT UNTO ABEL AND TO HIS OFFERING."*[43] But curiously enough, Cain, who was a strict vegetarian and "a tiller of the ground," offered up natural food's—fruit—to the Lord. *"BUT UNTO CAIN, AND TO HIS OFFERING, GOD HAD NO RESPECT."*[44] And because of these things did the latter fall into the power of the Devil. A mild warning to those who would engage themselves in a strict vegetarian diet alone!

However, the promised hope of the Millennium seems to bring a return of two things:

(a) a SECOND CHANGE in the physical appetite of man. "They shall not hurt nor destroy in all my holy mountain, saith the Lord."[45] Which would do away with animal slaughter for human consumption once and for all!

(b) a SECOND VISITATION by the Prophet of the Restoration. "I only go to return to you again,"[46] were his last remarks before that fateful march to Carthage.

Or, in other words, a return of Joseph Smith and natural foods!

NOTES

1 Leah D. Widstoe, *op., cit.*, p. 261.

2 *DUP Lesson for January*, 1968, p. 276 Kate B. Carter, compiler.

3. *Journal History*, August 16, 1846.

4. Frederick G. Williams Account Book, p. 237. Chuch Historian's Office, Salt Lake.

5. "Making Meals of Beans and Bread," by Nancy Albright; *Organic Gardening*, February, 1976, p. 144.

6. *Millennial Star* 93:149—150.

7. *Smith's Bible Dictionary*; Philadelphia, 1948, p. 544.

8. H.B. Tristam, *The Natural History of the Bible*; London, 1868, p. 47.

9. Daniel 1:20.

10. II Samuel 17:27—29.

11. Tristam, *op., cit.*

12. I Samuel 16:12.

13. *Joel Johnson Journal*, p. 29. No date, no place of publication. Church Library, Salt Lake.

14. *JD* 12:223.

15. Mosiah L. Hancock Journal, pp. 11-12, no date, no place of publication; Church Library, Salt Lake.

16. From a personal interview by the author, February, 1976.

17. *Deseret News*, Wednesday, January 29, 1975, p. 2A.

18. *Ibid.*, May 7, 1975, p. B9.

19. Hancock, *op., cit.*, pp. 14-15.

20. Deuteronomy 25:4.

21. *JD* 12:223.

22. *Deseret Weekly* 49:42

23 Brief History of Mary A Peterson, Roberta Clayton, *op., cit.,* fd. #122.

24. *JD* 15:78.

25. Autobiography of John L. Levy, p. 13; Utah Humanities Foundation, University of Utah.

26. *Ibid.*

27. N. B. Lundwall, *Faith Like The Ancients*, op. cit., p 68.

28. *Millennial Star*, 93:151.

29. Ivan J Barrett, *Joseph Smith and The Restoration*, p. 354.

30. W. A. Bennett, in a letter to *The Arizona Republican*, Phoenix, Arizona, November 17, 1932. Also to be found in Utah Humanities Foundation, Marriott Libraty, University of Utah.

31. *DHC* 5:549.

32. *DHC* 6:136.

33. *A String of Pearls*—Second Book of the Faith Promoting Series; Salt Lake City, 1880; p. 23.

34. *Journal of Heber McBride*, p. 6; Harold B. Lee Library, Special Collections, BYU.

35. *The New York Times*, Sunday, December 3, 1961.

36. *JD* 12:223.

37. Webster's *op. cit.*, p. 2632.

38. Widstoe. *op. cit.*, p.294.

39. *Ibid.*

40. *Ibid.*, pp. 294—295.

41. Genesis 2:18.

42. Genesis 1:31.

43. Genesis 5:7.

44. *Ibid.*

45. Isaiah 65:25.

46. Journal of Samuel H. Rogers, p. 201. Special Collections, BYU.

BIBLIOGRAPHY

Published Works

A String of Pearls—Second Book of The Faith-Promoting Series; Salt Lake, 1880.

Anderson, Nels, *Desert Saints;* Chicago, 1942.

Bancroft, Hubert Howe, *History of Utah.*

Barnes, Claude T., *The Grim Years*, Kaysville, Utah, 1964.

Barrett, Ivan J., *Joseph Smith and The Restoration.*

Braden, Clark and Kelly, E.L.; *Public Discussion of the Issues Between the Reorganized Church of Jesus Christ of Latter-day Saints and the Church of Christ disciples, held in Kirtland, Ohio;* St. Louis, 1884.

Burton, Richard F., *The City of The Saints;* New York, 1862.

BYU Studies

Cannon, George Q., *My First Mission—The First Book of The Faith-Promoting Series*; Salt Lake, 1882.

Carter, Kate B., *DUP Lessons.*

Cleland, Robert G. and Brooks, Juanita: *A Mormon Chronicle: The Diaries of John D. Lee;* San Marino, California, The Huntington Library, 1955.

Church News

Codman, John, *The Round Trip;* New York, 1879.

Colten, Mabel, *Biography of Elias H. Blackburn.*

Conference Report

Contributor

Crocheron, Augusta Joyce, *Representative Women of Deseret;* Salt Lake City, 1884.

Dall, Caroline H., *My first Holiday*; Boston, 1881.

Deseret News

Deseret Sunday Schools Songs, 1909.

Deseret Weekly

Dixon, Wm. Hepworth, *New America*; Philadelphia, 1867.

Doctrine & Covenants

Evans, John Henry, *Joseph Smith, An American Prophet*; New York, 1946.

Fife, Austin and Alta, *Saints of Sage & Saddle*; Indiana, 1956.

Frontier Guardian, Kanesville, Ohio.

Geddes, David D., *Health Aspects of the Word of Wisdom.*

Greeley, Horace, *An Overland Journey*; New York, 1864.

Harding, A.R., *Ginsing and Other Medicinal Plants*; Columbus, Ohio, 1936.

Heiser, Victor, *You're The Doctor*; New York, 1939.

Hill, Dr. Daniel B., *Hill Family History*; Salt Lake, 1927.

History of the Church

Hunter, Milton R.; *Beneath Ben Lomond's Peak.*

Improvement Era.

Ingersoll, Ernest, *The Crest of the Continent*; Chicago, 1885.

Inspired Version of the Holy Bible.

Jenson, Andrew, *Historical Record*; Salt Lake, 1886.

Johnson, Benjamin F., *My Life's Review*; Independence, Mo., 1947.

Johnson, Joel H., *A Voice From the Mountains.*

Jones, Daniel W., *Forty Years Among the Indians*; Salt Lake, 1890.

Journal of Discourses.

Juvenile Instructor.

Kane, Sarah Wood, *Twelve Mormon Homes Visited in Succession on a Journey Through Utah to Arizona*; Philadelphia, 1874.

LaWall, Charles H., *The Curious Lore of Drugs and Medicines (Four Thousand Years of Pharmacy);* New York, 1927.

Little, James A., *Jacob Hamblin, Fifth Book of the Faith-Promoting Series*; Salt Lake, 1881.

Lundwall, N.H., *Faith Like the Ancients*; Manti, 1973.

Mack, Solomon, *A Narrative of the Life of Solomon Mack;* Windsor, Vt., 1881.

McGavin, E. Cecil, *The Historical Background of the Doctrine and Covenants*; Salt Lake, 1949.

Millennial Star

Missouri Historical Society Bulletin; April, 1963.

Mulder, William and Mortensen, A. Russell; *Among the Mormons*; Lincoln, 1958.

Natural History Magazine, December, 1959.

New York Times, December 3, 1961.

Nibley, Preston, *Faith-Promoting Stories;* Missouri, 1943.

Organic Gardening.

Petersen, Paul H., *An Historical Analysis of the Word of Wisdom*; August, 1972, Master's thesis.

Petersen, LaMar, *Hearts Made Glad*; Salt Lake, 1975.

Pratt, Parley P., *Autobiography of Parley Parker Pratt*; New York, 1874.

Reader's Digest, May, 1945.

Remy, Jules and Julius Brenchley, *A Journey to Great Salt Lake City*; London, 1861.

Rodale, J.I.,. *The Encyclopedia of Organic Gardening*; Emmaus, Penn., December 1975.

Robinson, Ebenezer, "Items of Personal History of the Editor," *The Return*, I; Iowa, 1889.

Salt Lake Herald.

Schlink, F.J., *Eat, Drink, and Be Wary*; New York, 1935.

Smith, Eliza R. Snow, *Biography and Family Record of Lorenzo Snow*; Salt Lake, 1884.

Smith, Joseph Fielding, *Life of Joseph F. Smith*, Salt Lake, 1938.

Smith, Lucy Mack, *Joseph Smith and his Progenitors*; Lamoni, Iowa, 1912.

Smith, William, *Dictionary of the Bible*; Philadelphia, 1948.

Tagg, Melvin S., *The Life of Edward James Wood, Church Patriot*; July, 1959, Master's thesis.

Times and Seasons.

Tristam, H.B., *The Natural History of the Bible*; London, 1868.

Tullidge, Edward, *The Women of Mormondom*; New York, 1877.

United States Department of Agriculture Home and Garden Bulletin No. 72 *Nutritive Value of Foods*; Washington, D.C., January 1971.

Utah State Agricultural College, *Extension Bulletin*, No. 266, May 1953.

Webster's New International Dictionary of the English Language, Springfield, Mass., 1946.

Widtsoe, John A. and Leah D.; *The Word of Wisdom—A Modern Interpretation*; Salt Like City, 1937.

Widtsoe, Leah D., *How To Be Well*; Missouri, 1943.

Whitney, Orson F., *Whitney's Popular History of Utah.*

Wigington, Elliot., *Foxfire 3;* New York, 1975.

Woman's Exponent.

Young Men's Improvement Association Senior Manual, 1922-23.

Young Woman's Journal.

Archival Material

Abraham H. Cannon Journals, BYU.

Autobiography of Heber McBride, BYU. Amos Davis Account Book, University of Utah Library. Charles L. Walker Diary, BYU.

Diary of Emily Dow Partridge Young, BYU. Diary of L. John Nuttal, BYU.

Diary of Levi W. Hancock, BYU.

Evan Melbourne Greene Journal, CHO (Church Historian's Office).

Far West Record, CHO.

Frederick G. Williams Account Book, CHO.

History of the Life of Oliver B. Huntington, Church Library.

Journal History, Church Library.

John Heinerman's "Poems and Verses."

Joseph Smith's Journals, CHO.

Journals of Elder C.J. Hansen, BYU.

Journal of Edwin Harly, BYU.

Joel Johnson Journal, Church Library.

Journal of Jacob Hamblin, Utah State Historical Society.

Journal of Samuel H. Rogers, BYU.

Journal of William Henry Bigler, CHO.

Journal of S. Marsena Foster, University of Utah Library.

Kirtland High Council Minutes, CHO.

Lafayette C. Lee, "Reminiscences of Joseph Smith," BYU.

Lorenzo Brown Journal, BYU.

Mosiah L. Hancock Journal, Church Library.

Roberta Clayton Manuscript Collection, BYU.

Reiser, Arnold Auer Missionary Journal, BYU.

Utah Humanities Foundation Manuscript Collection, U of U Library.

William E. King Journals, CHO.

JOSEPH SMITH

AND

HERBAL MEDICINE

A Brief Study of The Botanic Arts in Mormonism

JOSEPH SMITH

AND ORGANIC LIFE

A Practical Guide to Successful Health

JOSEPH SMITH

AND THE COMING FAMINE

The Prophets on an Impending Crisis

JOSEPH SMITH FOR PRESIDENT

A Study of the Mormon Leader's Independent Party

0 26575 75030 0